Regional Antineoplastic Drug Delivery in the Management of Malignant Disease

The Johns Hopkins Series in Contemporary Medicine and Public Health

Regional Antineoplastic Drug Delivery in the Management of Malignant Disease

Maurie Markman, M.D.

Vice Chairman, Department of Medicine
Memorial Sloan-Kettering Cancer Center

The Johns Hopkins University Press
Baltimore and London

Notice: Readers should scrutinize product information sheets for dosage changes or contraindications, particularly for new or infrequently used drugs.

The Johns Hopkins University Press
701 West 40th Street
Baltimore, Maryland 21211
The Johns Hopkins Press Ltd., London

∞ The paper used in this book meets the minimum
requirements of American National Standards
for Information Sciences—Permanence of Paper
for Printed Library Materials, ANSI Z39.48-1984.

Library of Congress Cataloging-in-Publication Data

Markman, Maurie.
    Regional antineoplastic drug delivery in the management
of malignant disease / Maurie Markman.
        p.   cm. — (The Johns Hopkins series in
contemporary medicine and public health)
    Includes bibliographical references and index.
    ISBN 0-8018-4166-6 (alk. paper)
    1. Cancer—Chemotherapy.   2. Drug targeting.
3. Antineoplastic agents—Administration.   I. Title.
II. Series.
    [DNLM: 1. Antineoplastic Agents—administration &
dosage.   2. Antineoplastic Agents—therapeutic use.
3. Neoplasms—drug therapy.   QZ 267 M346r]
RC271.C5M27   1991
616.99'4061—dc20
DNLM/DLC
for Library of Congress   90-15596

To Tomi, Meg, Jon, Tim, and Betsey:
For all your love, I thank you.

Contents

Introduction

The principal aim of this book is to provide a state-of-the-art review of regional antineoplastic drug delivery in the management of malignant disease. Both the promise and the problems associated with the various forms of regional drug delivery that have been investigated at the clinical level are presented.

Despite more than 30 years of clinical research (Sullivan et al., 1953), most regional therapeutic techniques remain in the investigative sphere. Notable exceptions to this statement include prophylactic intrathecal cytotoxic drug delivery in the management of acute lymphocytic leukemia (Aur et al., 1971) and the intravesical delivery of antineoplastic agents as treatment of superficial bladder cancer (Soloway, 1984).

In the past decade, the establishment of improved surgical techniques, the development of new drug delivery systems, and the acquisition of a clearer understanding of the theoretical limitations and toxicities of regional therapy have enabled clinical researchers to embark on exciting new investigative programs in a number of areas involving regional antineoplastic drug delivery. These efforts range from the simple substitution of new drugs for established treatment indications (e.g., Bacillus Calmette-Guerin for intravesical treatment of superficial bladder cancer [Herr et al., 1988]) to highly experimental and innovative therapeutic concepts (e.g., direct intracavitary delivery of interleukin-2 and lymphokine-activated killer cells as treatment of malignant gliomas [Yoshida et al., 1988]).

I hope that individuals reading this book will come away with an understanding of where regional therapeutic approaches can be considered for standard patient management and where such therapy must, for the present, continue to be regarded as a potentially exciting investigative therapy. Although the scope of this book is limited to the regional drug delivery of antineoplastic agents, it is important to note that techniques of regional drug administration have been successfully employed in symptom management of patients with malignant disease, particularly in pain control (Payne, 1987).

The book is divided into seven chapters covering the major areas of clinical activity in regional antineoplastic drug delivery. These include regional vascular drug delivery in the management of tumor in the liver; intra-arterial therapy of malignant disease outside the liver; intraperitoneal therapy; intravesical therapy of superficial bladder cancer; and intrathecal treatment of leukemia, lymphoma, and meningeal carcinomatosis. In addition, an initial chapter briefly discusses some of the general principles of regional drug administration, and a final chapter presents a simple model whereby clinical investigators and health policymakers may examine the cost-effectiveness of a particular regional therapeutic technique relative to alternative treatment strategies.

Regional Antineoplastic Drug Delivery in the Management of Malignant Disease

1 General Principles of Regional Antineoplastic Drug Delivery

The principal goal of all forms of regional antineoplastic drug delivery is to increase the exposure of the tumor to the agent beyond the level that could safely be achieved by systemic drug administration (Collins, 1984) (Exhibit 1.1). Increased exposure of the drug to the tumor can be measured by an increase in peak drug levels attained in the region of the body containing the malignancy or by an increase in the area-under-concentration-versus-time curve (AUC).

The basic pharmacokinetic principles supporting regional drug delivery have been reviewed in detail by several authors (Chen and Gross, 1980; Collins, 1984; Dedrick et al., 1978; Markman, 1986; Sculier, 1985; Wolf and Sugarbaker, 1988).

The entire advantage of regional drug delivery results from the first pass of the agent through the perfused/infused area, even though the drug may

---

Exhibit 1.1

Aims of Regional Antineoplastic Drug Administration

- Increase exposure time to minimally/moderately active cytotoxic agents (both peak levels and total area-under-concentration-versus-time curve)

- Prolong the exposure of tumor to cycle-specific cytotoxic drugs

- Decrease systemic toxicity associated with intravenous therapy

- Enhance the opportunity to observe concentration-dependent synergy between two or more antineoplastic agents

---

Exhibit 1.2

Pharmacokinetic Advantage of Regional Drug Delivery

Equation 1:

$$R_{local} = C_{local}(regional) / C_{local}(IV).$$

Equation 2:

$$R_{systemic} = C_{systemic}(regional) / C_{systemic}(IV).$$

Equation 3:

$$R = \frac{R_{local}}{R_{systemic}} = \frac{C_{local}(regional) / C_{local}(IV)}{C_{systemic}(regional) / C_{systemic}(IV)}.$$

Note: R_{local} = relative increased exposure to infused/perfused region; $R_{systemic}$ = relative decreased exposure to systemic compartment; $C_{local}(regional)$ = local concentration following regional drug delivery; $C_{local}(IV)$ = local concentration following systemic drug delivery; $C_{systemic}(regional)$ = systemic concentration following local drug delivery; $C_{systemic}(IV)$ = systemic concentration following systemic drug delivery; R = overall pharmacokinetic advantage associated with regional drug delivery.

subsequently reach the target through the systemic circulation. Any pharmacokinetic advantage for regional exposure following local drug instillation is determined by comparing the amount of the drug delivered to the target area by this route of administration with the amount delivered by systemic delivery. Similarly, the extent of systemic exposure following regional treatment must be compared with that following intravenous drug administration to evaluate the relative advantage of the local approach in decreasing the amount of the drug entering the systemic compartment. It is possible to express these two concepts mathematically (see Equations 1 and 2 in Exhibit 1.2).

The overall advantage of regional drug delivery is defined as the ratio of the concentration reaching the perfused/infused region to the concentration reaching the systemic compartment (Equation 3 in Exhibit 1.2). Examination of Equation 3 in Exhibit 1.2 leads to one of the most important principles of regional therapy: The relative advantage of regional drug administration compared with systemic delivery will be significantly enhanced as regional drug clearance is reduced or systemic drug removal is increased.

Exhibit 1.3

Methods of Increasing the Pharmacokinetic Advantage Associated with Regional Drug Delivery

1. Removal of drug within the perfused organ (e.g., liver; Chapter 2);

2. Removal of drug following regional perfusion but prior to entry into systemic compartment (e.g., isolation–perfusion of extremities; Chapter 3);

3. Systemic delivery of an antagonist for the regionally administered cytotoxic drug to neutralize the agent and prevent systemic toxicity (e.g., leucovorin for methotrexate, thiosulfate for cisplatin; Chapter 4);

4. Use of a material to slow blood flow through the perfused organ (e.g., starch microspheres during liver perfusion; Chapter 2).

One can imagine a number of possible methods of increasing this regional advantage (Exhibit 1.3).

For example, drugs that are rapidly metabolized in the liver (i.e., have high systemic clearance) will exhibit the most favorable pharmacokinetic advantage following hepatic arterial, portal vein, or peritoneal cavity administration, because with these techniques of delivery drug uptake into the liver parenchyma will occur before the drug's entry into the systemic circulation.

Conversely, perfusion of a vessel or body cavity that does not lead to the removal of the active drug before its entry into the systemic compartment will, in general, be associated with a more limited pharmacokinetic advantage compared with intravenous administration. However, even without removal of the drug infused regionally there may be an advantage for this therapeutic approach if the blood flow through the region is sluggish and removal of the drug from the systemic compartment is rapid.

Even a modest increase in tumor–drug interactions may lead to an important increase in cytotoxicity if there is at least a modestly steep dose–response curve for the agent's activity against the tumor (Frei and Canellos, 1980). In addition, with minimal removal of the drug before its entry into the systemic circulation there will be less chance of a decrease in the therapeutic efficacy of the treament program due to a lower concentration of active drug reaching macroscopic or microscopic tumor outside the perfused region.

The toxicities associated with regional drug delivery can be both local and systemic. If the local toxic effects of an antineoplastic agent adminis-tered regionally are not dose limiting, it is possible to escalate the amount of the drug administered to the point where as much of the drug reaches the systemic compartment as when the agent is delivered intravenously (Howell et al., 1982; Stewart et al., 1983). Thus, the extent of systemic exposure following regional drug delivery will depend to a large degree on the drug(s) used and the specific route(s) of drug administration employed.

It is important to appreciate that, in general, any advantage of regional drug administration over systemic drug delivery will be relative, rather than absolute. Limited experimental data support the concept that there will be a modest increase in tissue and tumor drug concentration locally following regional drug administration (Carlson et al., 1984; Los et al., 1989; Stewart, Benjamin, et al., 1982; Stewart et al., 1988; Stewart, Leavens, et al., 1982; Vennin et al., 1989). Thus, it can be anticipated that regional drug delivery may enhance the activity of antineoplastic agents with known effectiveness (even if only marginal) against a particular tumor type, but will be incapable of converting a totally inactive drug into a highly active cytotoxic agent.

Finally, when evaluating the relative effectiveness of a regional therapy program compared with an alternative systemic approach, it is important to consider both the cost (in funds, personnel, and morbidity) of the procedure and the overall clinical benefit. In addition, regional therapeutic approaches will usually require greater technical expertise (surgical and medical) and have the potential for greater morbidity than standard intravenous therapy. This point must be kept in mind whenever an individual physician or insti-tution plans to initiate a regional antineoplastic treatment program.

2 Regional Vascular Drug Delivery for Malignant Disease Confined to the Liver

2.1 Scope of the clinical issues and alternative treatment options

Because the greatest experience with regional antineoplastic therapy for tumor in the liver has been with treatment of metastatic colon carcinoma, this chapter focuses on that topic. Hepatic arterial therapy for other tumor types is briefly discussed in Section 2.9.

Approximately one hundred fifty thousand individuals were found to have developed colorectal carcinoma in the United States in 1989 (Silverberg and Lubera, 1989). Sixty thousand of these patients died of their disease, and at least 20 to 30 percent of these deaths were the direct result of metastatic tumor in the liver (Hanks and Jones, 1986; Welch and Donaldson, 1979). The overall median survival of patients with untreated liver metastases from colon carcinoma is approximately 5 months (Bengtsson et al., 1981). However, survival is greatly influenced by the extent of liver involvement at the time of diagnosis and can range from as short a period of time as 3 months (for widespread tumor in the liver) to as long as 17 months (for solitary lesions) (Wood, Gillis, and Blumgart, 1976).

The only known curative treatment strategy for patients with metastatic colon carcinoma in the liver is surgical resection of the tumor (Adson and Van Heerdon, 1980; Fortner et al., 1984; Niederhuber and Ensminger, 1983). Unfortunately, it has been estimated that only 5 to 10 percent of all patients with colon carcinoma metastatic to the liver are appropriate candidates for a curative surgical approach (Niederhuber and Ensminger, 1983).

Since the 1950s, 5-fluorouracil (5-FU) has been the single most active and important drug in the management of metastatic colon carcinoma, including metastatic disease in the liver (Kemeny, 1983, 1987). The response rate of metastatic colon carcinoma to 5-FU has varied in different series from 10 to 25 percent. Unfortunately, almost all responses are only partial

5

and the duration of response is generally short (less than 6 to 8 months). 5-Fluorouracil-based chemotherapy has improved the response rate of colon carcinoma in several series, but the impact of such therapy on overall survival has not been significant (Kemeny, 1987). The recent addition of leucovorin to 5-FU as treatment of metastatic colon carcinoma has increased the response rate of metastatic colon carcinoma into the 30 to 45 percent range, but an overall survival benefit in metastatic disease has yet to be convincingly demonstrated (Grem et al., 1987; Poon et al., 1989).

One of the major difficulties encountered when attempting to compare treatment programs for patients with metastatic colon carcinoma in the liver and determine whether a specific regimen has favorably influenced survival is the known overriding impact of the extent of liver involvement at the time of treatment initiation in defining ultimate patient outcome. For example, in a large series of patients with metastatic colon carcinoma confined to the liver reported from the Memorial Sloan-Kettering Cancer Center, patients with 30 percent or less liver involvement with tumor had a median survival of 24 months compared with a 10-month median survival for those individuals with greater than 30 percent involvement (Kemeny, Niedzwiecki, et al., 1989).

2.2 Rationale for regional drug delivery in the management of patients with colon carcinoma metastatic to the liver

As with other forms of regional treatment of malignant disease, the principal goal of either hepatic arterial or portal vein infusional therapy of colon carcinoma metastatic to the liver is to expose the tumor in that organ to higher concentrations of the antineoplastic agent(s) for longer time periods than can be achieved with systemic drug delivery. At the same time it is hoped that systemic toxicity can be reduced. In theory, prolonged exposure of tumor to a chemotherapeutic agent is a particularly important advantage for cycle-specific drugs such as 5-FU and fluorodeoxyuridine (FUDR) (Chabner et al., 1975).

The liver is the ideal organ to perfuse with cytotoxic drugs because several of the commonly used antineoplastic agents, including 5-FU and FUDR, are rapidly and extensively metabolized into nontoxic metabolites during their first passage through the liver (Ensminger et al., 1978).

Because the liver has a duel blood supply (portal vein and hepatic artery), it is important that the regional infusion be delivered into the vascular compartment actually supplying the tumor. Several preclinical and clinical studies have now firmly established that macroscopic tumor in the liver (nodules greater than 1 to 2 mm in diameter) receives its blood supply principally (95 percent or more) from the hepatic artery (Ackerman, 1974; Bierman et al., 1951; Breedis and Young, 1954; Conway, Popp, and Thurman, 1985; Daly et al., 1987; Lien and Ackerman, 1970; Lin et al., 1984; Ridge et al., 1987; Sigurdson et al., 1987; Solt, Hoy, and Farber, 1977). In contrast, the normal liver receives 75 to 80 percent of its blood supply from the portal vein, with the remainder coming from the hepatic artery (Bierman et al., 1951).

In a recent study investigators at the Memorial Sloan-Kettering Cancer Center sampled tumor and normal tissue following either hepatic artery or portal vein infusions of FUDR. The mean drug levels in normal cells did not differ significantly depending on the route of drug delivery. However, the mean tumor levels following hepatic artery infusions were more than 15 times higher than that found when the same dose of FUDR was delivered via the portal vein (Sigurdson et al., 1987).

In addition, in a small randomized trial from the same institution comparing hepatic arterial with portal venous infusions of FUDR, 4 of 8 patients receiving therapy by the arterial route responded compared with none of 11 individuals treated by direct delivery into the portal vein (Daly et al., 1987). Nine of these latter patients crossed over to hepatic arterial therapy and 3 experienced objective tumor regressions. Finally, at least one report has suggested that the prognosis following hepatic artery ligation and regional chemotherapy in patients with metastatic colon carcinoma in the liver is directly related to tumor vascularity as demonstrated on angiogram (Kim et al., 1977).

In contrast to the overwhelming data suggesting the superiority of the hepatic arterial route for regional therapy of established macroscopic colon carcinoma present in the liver, there exists a strong rationale for considering portal vein infusions as therapy of microscopic tumor in the liver. Several experimental observations support this argument. First, a number of investigators have demonstrated that microscopic colon carcinoma present in the liver receives at least 50 percent of its blood supply from the portal vein (Conway, Popp, and Thurman, 1983; Lin et al., 1984). In addition, in situations where the blood supply to macroscopic tumor from the hepatic artery is disrupted (i.e., hepatic artery ligation or thrombosis), the portal circulation appears to be capable of providing adequate nutrient delivery to maintain viable tumor (Ackerman, 1986; Flowerdew et al., 1987; Lien and Ackerman, 1970). This phenomenon may explain why total occlusion of the hepatic artery does not necessarily prevent tumor growth in the liver.

At this point it is important that one theoretical concern with regional vascular drug delivery in general and hepatic arterial administration in particular be addressed. Most investigators considering intra-arterial therapy as a therapeutic option have assumed that this route of drug delivery results in a homogeneous distribution of drug throughout the perfused region (Dedrick, 1988). However, recent experimental data have seriously questioned this assumption because it has been shown that severe "streaming effects" observed at flow rates achieved within the hepatic artery following drug perfusion result in nonuniform drug distribution to the perfused tissue (Lutz and Miller, 1988). It is unknown at present what role, if any, this experimental observation plays in the known variability of response in patients treated by direct regional vascular antineoplastic drug administration to the liver and other body sites.

2.3 Early clinical experience with hepatic arterial therapy for colon carcinoma metastatic to the liver

The initial trials of delivering chemotherapeutic agents directly into the hepatic artery as treatment for colon carcinoma metastatic to the liver were reported in the 1950s and 1960s (Clarkson et al., 1962; Klopp et al., 1950; Sullivan et al., 1953). In several large series of patients treated through the 1970s, an overall objective response or clinical improvement rate of 40 to 70 percent was observed (Ansfield and Ramirez, 1978; Buroker et al., 1976; Cady and Oberfield, 1974; Tandon, Bunnell, and Cooper, 1973).

Unfortunately, there are a number of problems with these early reports. First, the definition of response and/or clinical improvement was not standardized and often quite subjective. Second, the impact of this therapeutic approach on survival, despite the extremely high response rates reported, is questionable (Bedikian, 1983). Comparison of survival of patients treated by hepatic arterial infusion therapy with those managed by systemic antineoplastic drug delivery is made difficult by the fact that most individuals treated by the regional approach had disease clinically limited to the liver and selection bias may have played a major role in any perceived survival benefit for hepatic arterial therapy (Huberman, 1983).

Finally, the early trials of hepatic artery drug delivery frequently relied on percutaneous catheter placement (under angiographic guidance) to deliver only one or several treatment courses. This limited the number of treatments possible and often the duration of each treatment course. As noted above, prolonged exposure to cycle-specific drugs may be important in achieving maximal benefit from this route of drug delivery. In addition, the complications associated with this approach were often excessive and in-cluded arterial thrombosis, catheter dislodgement (leading to significant drug delivery to the gastrointestinal mucosa), and infection (Huberman, 1983; Niederhuber and Ensminger, 1983; Oberfield, 1983a; Sterchi, 1985). Also, with percutaneously placed hepatic arterial catheters, prolonged hos-pitalizations (up to 10 days) were required for each treatment course.

2.4 The implantable pump for hepatic arterial chemotherapy

In the late 1970s, implantable continuous infusion systems for hepatic artery drug delivery became available (Barone, 1986; Buchwald et al., 1980; Ens-minger et al., 1981; Niederhuber and Ensminger, 1983). The surgical tech-niques recommended for catheter placement have been extensively dis-cussed elsewhere and are not reviewed here (Albano et al., 1984; Chu, Hutchins, and Lang, 1988; Daly et al., 1984; Niederhuber and Ensminger, 1983; Sterchi, 1985; Williams and Daly, 1989).

However, one important point relevant to both the surgery performed to insert the hepatic artery catheter and subsequent chemotherapy administra-tion should be noted. Following the delivery of chemotherapeutic agents into the hepatic artery, the gallbladder is exposed to extremely high concentra-tions of the infused drugs, because in 95 percent of individuals the cystic artery is a branch of the hepatic artery. Therefore, it is not surprising that acute cholecystitis has been commonly observed in patients receiving he-patic arterial chemotherapy through long-term infusion devices (Hohn et al., 1986; Lafon, Reed, and Rosenthal, 1985; Ottery, Scupham, and Weese, 1986). As a result, cholecystectomy is now recommended at the time of surgical catheter placement for all patients receiving an implantable hepatic artery catheter.

2.5 Recent clinical experience with hepatic arterial therapy for colon carcinoma metastatic to the liver employing implantable infusion devices

In contrast to the earlier experience with percutaneously placed hepatic ar-terial catheters, when 5-FU was the single agent most commonly selected for treatment, recent studies using the implantable catheters have usually employed FUDR. This is due to the fact that whereas 20 to 50 percent of the 5-FU is extracted during its first passage through the liver, 95 to 99 percent of the FUDR is removed. Thus, the pharmacokinetic advantage

---

Exhibit 2.1

**Most Extensively Investigated Program for Hepatic Arterial
Therapy for Colon Cancer Metastatic to the Liver**

---

1. Surgical placement of a hepatic arterial catheter;
2. Fluorodeoxyuridine (0.3 mg/kg/day) by continuous infusion for 14 days;
3. Following a 14-day break, reinstitution of treatment;
4. Continuation of treatment in responding patients (assuming acceptable toxicity) until the disease progresses.

(and limitation of systemic exposure and toxicity) associated with the hepatic arterial infusion of FUDR is superior to that of 5-FU (Ensminger and Gyves, 1983; Ensminger et al., 1978).

A number of Phase 2 trials of hepatic arterial infusional therapy of colon carcinoma metastatic to the liver employing FUDR delivered through a surgically implanted delivery device have been reported. The most commonly used regimen has been continuous infusion of FUDR at a rate of 0.3 mg/kg/day for 14 days (Exhibit 2.1) (Stagg et al., 1984). Following a 2-week break, treatment is restarted. In general, treatment is continued until disease progression or unacceptable toxicity develops.

Unfortunately, the criteria for a patient to be said to have achieved a response have varied considerably in the various reported series. Whereas some studies employed standard criteria for a partial response (Miller et al., 1981), others accepted a fall in carcinoembryonic antigen only as evidence of an antitumor effect. Overall, approximately 40 to 60 percent of previously untreated patients with colon carcinoma metastatic to the liver have been shown to respond to hepatic arterial infusional therapy with FUDR (Kemeny et al., 1984; Stagg et al., 1984; Van de Velde et al., 1988; Weiss et al., 1983), although individual studies have reported response rates as low as 15 percent (Schwartz, 1984) and as high as 83 to 88 percent (Balch et al., 1983; Niederhuber et al., 1984). Responses are also observed in approximately 15 to 25 percent of patients previously treated with systemic chemotherapy, including 5-FU (Kemeny et al., 1984; Stagg et al., 1984).

As noted above, it is difficult to make any definitive statement about the impact of hepatic arterial therapy on survival on the basis of these Phase 2 trials because this important end point will be greatly influenced by the degree of liver involvement when treatment is initiated (Kemeny et al.,

1984; Kemeny, Niedzwiecki, et al., 1989; Patt et al., 1986). Several authors have attempted to examine the overall impact of hepatic arterial therapy on survival by comparing the clinical results of nonrandomized patients treated either by this route of drug delivery or by systemic drug administration. Not surprisingly, these reports have either suggested this therapeutic approach is associated with a survival benefit for patients treated in this manner (Balch et al., 1983; Niederhuber et al., 1984), or stated that the observed higher response rate with regional therapy results in no or only a marginal impact on survival (Bedikian et al., 1984; Weiss et al., 1983).

2.6 Randomized controlled trials of hepatic arterial therapy for colon carcinoma metastatic to the liver

In general, it is only through the conduct of carefully designed randomized clinical trials that the overall impact of a new treatment strategy can be critically evaluated. These trials must control for the known important prognostic factors in a disease, including extent of tumor involvement, patient performance status, and prior treatment. Several randomized trials comparing hepatic arterial therapy with systemic drug delivery as therapy for colon carcinoma metastatic to the liver have been reported either in preliminary form or as final reports.

The Central Oncology Group randomized 74 patients with colon carcinoma metastatic to the liver to either hepatic arterial or systemic 5-FU. There was no difference in response rate, time to disease progression, or survival in the two treatment groups (Grage et al., 1979). Interpretation of the results of this trial is made difficult by the fact that patients treated by the hepatic arterial route received only 21 days of regional therapy with 5-FU (14 days at 20 mg/kg/day followed by 7 days at 10 mg/kg/day). These patients were then maintained on weekly intravenous 5-FU. It can certainly be argued that a single 21-day course of hepatic arterial therapy is insufficient to significantly affect the clinical course of patients with metastatic disease in the liver.

Investigators at the National Cancer Institute treated a group of 64 patients with colon carcinoma metastatic to the liver with either hepatic arterial FUDR (0.3 mg/kg/day for 14 days) or intravenous FUDR (Chang et al., 1987). The response rate to drug delivered regionally (62 percent) was significantly higher ($p < 0.003$) than that observed with systemic drug administration (17 percent). Unfortunately, by actuarial analysis, there was no overall impact on survival, with 22 percent and 15 percent of patients treated with hepatic or intravenous infusions, respectively, surviving for 2 years.

When patients with positive hepatic lymph nodes were excluded from the analysis, a survival advantage for regional drug delivery was suggested.

Investigators at the Memorial Sloan-Kettering Cancer Center conducted a randomized trial of hepatic arterial FUDR (0.3 mg/kg/day for 14 days) versus continuous intravenous FUDR (0.15 mg/kg/day for 14 days) (Kemeny, 1987). Patients progressing on the systemic drug arm were allowed to cross over to the regional drug regimen. The response rate to hepatic arterial therapy (50 percent) was significantly higher ($p < 0.001$) than that observed following systemic drug delivery (20 percent). Although there was no overall impact on survival observed between the two treatment programs, it should be noted that 60 percent of the patients progressing on the systemic arm crossed over to receive hepatic arterial FUDR, 25 percent of whom achieved a partial remission. This "secondary response" may have significantly improved the overall survival of the patient population randomized to the systemic treatment and obscured a potential survival benefit for regional drug delivery.

In the Sloan-Kettering trial, extrahepatic disease developed in 56 percent and 37 percent of patients receiving hepatic arterial and intravenous therapy, respectively. Although this difference was of only borderline statistical significance, it suggests that whereas control of disease in the liver may be improved with regional drug delivery, disease progression outside the liver can be anticipated because of the limited systemic drug exposure to FUDR following hepatic arterial infusion.

The Northern California Oncology Group conducted a randomized trial of hepatic arterial or systemic therapy of colon carcinoma metastatic to the liver that was similar in design to the Sloan-Kettering study noted above, except that the doses of hepatic arterial (0.2 mg/kg/day) and intravenous (0.075 mg/kg/day) FUDR were lower than in the Sloan-Kettering trial (Hohn et al., 1989). The initial dose of hepatic arterial FUDR employed in this trial was 0.3 mg/kg/day, but because 10 of the first 25 patients treated on the trial developed radiographic evidence of biliary strictures the dose was reduced. A total of 143 patients were entered into this study. Responses were demonstrated in 42 percent of patients receiving hepatic arterial therapy compared with only 10 percent of individuals treated by the systemic route of drug delivery.

In the Mayo Clinic/North Central Cancer Treatment Group trial, 74 patients with colon carcinoma metastatic to the liver were randomized to receive either hepatic arterial FUDR (0.3 mg/kg/day for 14 days) or intravenous 5-FU (500 mg/m² push Days 1 to 5 every 5 weeks) (O'Connell et al., 1989). This study differed from the Sloan-Kettering and Northern California

Oncology Group trials in that a crossover from systemic to hepatic arterial therapy was not permitted at the time of disease progression. The response to regional drug therapy (54 percent) was significantly higher ($p < 0.01$) than that observed with intravenous treatment (21 percent), but there was no overall impact on survival ($p = 0.44$). In addition, whereas the median time to progression in the liver following hepatic arterial drug administration (14 months) was significantly longer than that observed with systemic therapy (7 months), the overall time to progression was not different between the two treatment arms.

Finally, a randomized trial reported from the City of Hope National Medical Center examined the possible clinical utility of hepatic arterial therapy in patients undergoing surgical resection of liver metastases from colon carcinoma, as well as in those individuals with unresectable lesions (Kemeny et al., 1986). Patients with solitary metastatic nodules were randomized to undergo surgery only or surgery with hepatic arterial therapy with FUDR. Patients with multiple resectable metastatic lesions were randomized to regional chemotherapy alone or chemotherapy plus surgery. Patients with unresectable metastatic tumor in the liver were randomized to hepatic arterial therapy with FUDR or intravenous 5-FU. In this trial there was a suggestion that patients undergoing resection of multiple metastatic lesions in the liver (along with regional drug delivery) may have experienced superior survival compared with those individuals treated with chemotherapy alone.

This study, as well as others (Hodgson et al., 1986), supports the aggressive treatment of patients with metastatic colon carcinoma in the liver with a combined surgical/regional chemotherapy approach. However, the ultimate impact of such therapy in this clinical setting can be defined only in larger randomized trials specifically designed to examine this issue. Unfortunately, even if disease is controlled in the liver, with the currently available chemotherapeutic agents it is likely the cancer will progress in extrahepatic sites.

2.7 Toxicity of hepatic arterial therapy with fluorodeoxyuridine

Because of the extensive extraction of FUDR during its first passage through the liver, systemic exposure is limited and systemic side effects are usually very mild following hepatic arterial delivery (Hohn et al., 1986; Kemeny, Daly, et al., 1987). In contrast, serious morbidity secondary to the high local arterial concentrations of FUDR bathing the liver has been observed (Daly et al., 1987; Doria et al., 1986; Hohn et al., 1986; Hohn, Melnick, et al., 1985; Kemeny et al., 1984, 1985; Kemeny, Daly, et al., 1987; Shepard et al., 1987).

It has been hypothesized that gastric and duodenal inflammation noted following hepatic arterial infusions of FUDR, which ultimately leads to ulcerations, is due to misdirection of the infused FUDR into the right gastric artery and other smaller vessels leading to the stomach (Hohn, Stagg, et al., 1985; Narsete et al., 1977). The incidence of gastric irritation reported in different series has varied from 0 to 50 percent. This striking difference likely reflects the diligence with which the various investigators have sought to diagnose asymptomatic patients (i.e., endoscopy), and surgeons have attempted to ligate vessels feeding the stomach at the time of hepatic arterial catheter placement. One report has suggested that the clinical problem of gastric ulceration can be almost totally eliminated if meticulous care is taken at the time of catheter implantation to identify vessels distal to the catheter that lead to the duodenum and stomach (Hohn, Stagg, et al., 1985).

Chemical hepatitis has been reported to occur in as many as 96 percent of patients treated with hepatic arterial FUDR if elevations in liver enzymes alone are considered to be evidence of hepatic irritation (Hohn et al., 1986; Hohn, Melnick, et al., 1985). In most patients the enzyme elevations return to normal with discontinuation or interruption of treatment (Daly et al., 1987; Shepard et al., 1987).

However, a more serious complication of treatment is the development of sclerosing cholangitis or biliary sclerosis, which may or may not be reversible and can ultimately lead to the patient's death (Kemeny et al., 1985). Biliary sclerosis has been reported to occur in 8 to 20 percent of patients treated with hepatic arterial FUDR (Hohn et al., 1986; Hohn, Melnick, et al., 1985; Kemeny, Daly, et al., 1987; Kemeny et al., 1985; Pettavel et al., 1988). Of interest, the study reporting the lowest incidence of gastric toxicity with hepatic arterial FUDR had the highest incidence of biliary toxicity, suggesting that success in ligating vessels feeding the stomach increases the exposure of the liver to the chemotherapeutic agent (Hohn et al., 1986; Hohn, Melnick, et al., 1985).

The liver demonstrates a number of pathologic features when patients develop hepatic toxicity secondary to hepatic arterial infusions of FUDR. These include necrosis of hepatocytes, cholestasis, steatosis, central vein sclerosis, and portal triad and micronodular cirrhosis (Doria et al., 1986). In patients with biliary sclerosis, cholangiography will demonstrate both intrahepatic and extrahepatic bile duct sclerosis (Hohn, Melnick, et al., 1985; Kemeny et al., 1985).

Two recent reports have suggested that corticosteroids may markedly reduce the severity of hepatic arterial chemotherapy-induced cholestatic jaundice (Janis, Leming, and Leder, 1988; Seiter et al., 1990). This interesting and potentially important preliminary observation will need to be confirmed in larger clinical trials.

2.8 Other single-agent and combination chemotherapy programs using the hepatic arterial route as therapy for colon carcinoma metastatic to the liver

Although single-agent 5-FU or FUDR is the most common treatment regimen reported for hepatic arterial therapy of metastatic colon carcinoma in the liver, investigators at several centers have examined alternative treatment programs. Included in the list of reported regimens are single-agent mitomycin C (Schneider et al., 1989); sequential 5-FU and FUDR (Stagg et al., 1984); FUDR or 5-FU and mitomycin C (Cohen, Kaufman, and Wood, 1984; Donegan, 1985; Patt et al., 1980; Shepard et al., 1985); FUDR, mitomycin, and N,N'-bis (2-chloro-ethyl)-N-nitrosourea (BCNU) (Cohen, Schaeffer, and Higgins, 1986); FUDR and cisplatin (Patt et al., 1986); FUDR or 5-FU with mitomycin and doxorubicin (Khayat et al., 1988; Pfeifle, Howell, and Bookstein, 1985); and FUDR with leucovorin (Kemeny, Cohen, et al., 1989). Although objective responses have been observed with the use of all of these regimens, there is no convincing evidence that any combination program for hepatic arterial therapy of colon carcinoma metastatic to the liver is superior to single-agent FUDR.

Two of the aforementioned trials are worthy of further mention. In a recently reported study from the Memorial Sloan-Kettering Cancer Center, 78 patients with metastatic colon carcinoma involving the liver were treated with hepatic arterial mitomycin C after failure of hepatic arterial FUDR or after removal of this treatment program secondary to toxicity (Schneider et al., 1989). Mitomycin C was administered at a dose of 10 mg/m_2 every 4 to 6 weeks. Eleven of 64 patients (17 percent) responded, with the major toxicity reported being bone marrow suppression. Hepatic arterial mitomycin C infusion would seem to be a reasonable treatment option in patients who cannot receive FUDR because of excessive hepatic toxicity.

In the second report from Sloan-Kettering, patients with colon carcinoma metastatic to the liver were treated with FUDR plus leucovorin (Kemeny, Cohen, et al., 1989). The major justification for this trial was the previously reported preclinical and clinical data suggesting pronounced synergy between these two drugs in the treatment of colon carcinoma (Grem et al., 1987). Although considerable local toxicity was encountered (enzyme elevations and biliary sclerosis) in the initial trial, a high objective response rate (greater than 60 percent) was noted in a small number of patients included in the initial preliminary report.

2.9 Hepatic arterial therapy for other tumor types

There are a number of published reports from investigators treating both primary hepatocellular carcinomas and a variety of noncolon carcinomas metastatic to the liver with hepatic arterial infusions of cytotoxic drugs (Ajani et al., 1989; Calvo et al., 1980; Doci et al., 1988; Khayat et al., 1988; Malone et al., 1987; Malvigit et al., 1988; O'Connell et al., 1988; Patt et al., 1988; Stehlin et al., 1988; Weiss et al., 1983). Included among the metastatic tumor types evaluated are islet cell tumors; carcinoids; melanomas; and breast, anal, gallbladder, bile duct, and ovarian cancer. Although responses have been observed, the impact of such treatment on overall survival is uncertain.

In one recent report, the median survival of patients with hepatoma treated with hepatic arterial therapy (either 5-FU or doxorubicin) was only 3.5 months (Doci et al., 1988). However, responders lived significantly longer than nonresponders: 13 months versus 2 months, respectively. Similar data have been reported by investigators at the M. D. Anderson Hospital (Patt et al., 1988).

2.10 Innovative treatment programs involving the hepatic arterial route of drug delivery

Investigators at a number of centers have attempted to improve the efficacy of therapy for primary hepatic tumors and metastatic cancer in the liver by developing innovative therapeutic techniques employing the hepatic arterial route. Several of these approaches are briefly summarized below.

One of the major limitations of hepatic arterial therapy is the fact that rapid blood flow through the vessel decreases the exposure time of the tumor to the infused drug. Short-term blockade of the hepatic arterial blood supply with material degradable by hepatic enzymes (i.e., starch and ethylcellulose) allows for increased uptake of drug into the surrounding tumor tissue, while also allowing for increased time for the drug to be metabolized in the liver (Thom et al., 1989; Wilmott, 1987). This technique, sometimes called *chemoembolization,* would be of particular relevance for drugs, such as mitomycin C (Hu and Howell, 1983), that are not rapidly cleared from the blood during their first passage through the hepatic circulation (Ensminger et al., 1985; Pfeifle et al., 1986), but it has also been demonstrated to increase tumor exposure to agents that are extensively metabolized in the liver, including FUDR and doxorubicin (Pfeifle et al., 1986; Sigurdson, Ridge, and Daly, 1986; Thom et al., 1989). As with other innovative programs employing the regional route of drug delivery, it remains uncertain whether responses observed with this therapeutic approach are superior to those following administration of the chemotherapeutic agents without the temporary blockade of hepatic arterial blood flow (Dakhil et al., 1982; Ichihara et al., 1989; Patt et al., 1981; Pfeifle, Howell, and Bookstein, 1985; Wilmott, 1987; Wollner et al., 1986).

Another approach to increase the concentration of the drug reaching the tumor while decreasing systemic exposure is *isolation perfusion* of the liver. The goal of this technique, which has been examined both experimentally (Ghussen, Nagel, and Isselhard, 1983) and in limited clinical trials (Aigner, 1988; Schalhorn, Peyerl, and Denecke, 1988), is to completely isolate the blood supply of the liver from the systemic circulation while the organ is being perfused with high concentrations of the chemotherapeutic agent. This is a technically demanding procedure whose ultimate role in patient management remains to be defined (Schalhorn, Peyerl, and Denecke, 1988).

The hepatic arterial administration of radioisotopes along with microspheres that transiently reduce blood flow and increase tumor exposure to the ionizing radiation has been examined in a Phase 1 and 2 trial using yttrium-90 (Boos et al., 1989; Herba et al., 1988). Using this approach, it was possible to locally deliver up to 10,000 cGy with acceptable local and systemic toxicities.

Investigators at the National Cancer Institute recently reported on a Phase 1 trial of the hepatic arterial infusion of iododeoxyuridine in patients with metastatic colon carcinoma (Chang et al., 1989). The drug was delivered by continuous infusion for 14 days. Of considerable interest, antitumor activity was observed and there was no evidence of hepatic toxicity. There was also evidence of incorporation of the agent preferentially into the DNA of tumor cells. Finally, iododeoxyuridine has been demonstrated experimentally to be the radiosensitizing agent and the potential exists for increased therapeutic efficacy of external radiotherapy when delivered following regional administration of the agent. A related compound, 5-bromo-2'-deoxyuridine, has similar properties that also make it an attractive agent for hepatic arterial administration (Ensminger, 1989).

Investigators in Japan have examined the clinical utility of hepatic arterial cisplatin administered along with systemically delivered thiosulfate to protect against cisplatin-induced nephrotoxicity (Abe et al., 1988). (The rationale supporting this therapeutic approach is described in detail in Section 4.5.4 in Chapter 4.)

Hepatic arterial chemotherapy for colon carcinoma metastatic to the liver followed by consolidation with external radiation has been examined by investigators at the Cleveland Clinic (Miller et al., 1988). Unfortunately, despite an acceptable toxicity profile, there was no evidence of increased efficacy compared with hepatic arterial therapy alone.

Hepatic arterial cisplatin suspended in an oily lymphographic agent has been evaluated as therapy for hepatocellular carcinoma (Shibata et al., 1989). The lymphographic agent had previously been demonstrated to selectively accumulate in hepatoma cells following local instillation. In a recently reported clinical trial, platinum concentrations in tumor tissues were found to be 40 times higher than in nonmalignant tissue. The 1-year survival rate of 55 percent was somewhat encouraging. Further exploration of this approach appears indicated.

2.11 Adjuvant therapy of colon carcinoma employing the portal vein route of drug delivery

As previously discussed (Section 2.2), preclinical and clinical data fail to support the use of portal vein infusions as therapy for established macroscopic metastatic colon carcinoma present in the liver. However, treatment of microscopic disease in the liver by portal vein infusions in the adjuvant setting might be appropriate in patients undergoing resection of the primary colon lesion, who have a high risk of developing recurrent disease.

A randomized trial from England examining the clinical utility of adjuvant portal vein infusions of 5-FU in patients with colon carcinoma has suggested this treatment approach decreases the risk of the development of hepatic metastases and improves overall survival (Taylor, Brooman, and Rowling, 1977; Taylor et al., 1985; Taylor, Rowling, and West, 1979). Although of considerable interest, these results are somewhat surprising because the specific treatment program employed in this trial consisted of only a single 7-day course of portal vein 5-FU (1 g/day by continuous infusion) immediately following surgery.

Several groups are currently attempting to confirm the findings of the English study. Of the three preliminary reports, two appear to support the basic conclusion that adjuvant portal vein therapy is of benefit in patients with colon carcinoma (Metzger et al., 1989; Wolmark et al., 1990), while the third trial was unable to establish any benefit for this therapeutic maneuver (Ryan et al., 1988). For the present, adjuvant portal vein infusional therapy for colon carcinoma must be considered an interesting experimental approach whose ultimate impact on survival of patients with colon carcinoma remains to be determined.

2.12 Summary and recommendations

Several general conclusions can appropriately be reached regarding the current status of hepatic arterial therapy for colon carcinoma metastatic to the liver (also see Exhibits 2.2 and 2.3):

1. Objective response rates to hepatic arterial FUDR infusions in patients previously untreated with chemotherapy are approximately double (40 to 50 percent) those that can be achieved with systemically delivered FUDR or 5-FU (15 to 20 percent).

Exhibit 2.2

Fluorodeoxyuridine by Hepatic Arterial Infusion as Treatment of Colorectal Cancer Metastatic to the Liver

Overall objective response rate: 40–50 percent

Overall median survival: 15–20 months

Major toxicity: gastritis, ulcer, chemical hepatitis, biliary sclerosis

---

Exhibit 2.3

Hepatic Arterial versus Intravenous Therapy for Liver Metastases from Colon Cancer: Reasonable Conclusions from the Results of Comparative Trials

1. Hepatic arterial therapy results in a doubling of the objective response rate compared with intravenous treatment.
2. There is no significant impact of regional therapy on overall survival in this clinical setting.
3. Patients who fail systemic treatment may subsequently respond to hepatic arterial therapy with fluorodeoxyuridine.
4. Hepatic arterial therapy is an acceptable initial treatment option for appropriately selected patients, particularly those whose major symptoms are due to the presence of tumor in the liver.

2. Although these responses may be translated into improved symptom control and quality of life for patients treated in this manner (see Chapter 7), there is as yet no convincing evidence that this therapeutic approach is associated with a survival benefit compared with treatment by the systemic route of drug delivery (Van De Velde et al., 1988).

3. Although improvements in regional drug administration (i.e., combination FUDR plus leucovorin) may increase the objective response rate in the liver and prevent disease progression in this organ, it is unlikely that such therapy will have any major overall impact on survival of patients with metastatic colon carcinoma until improved methods are found to control systemic disease progression. Unfortunately, a recently reported small randomized trial of hepatic arterial FUDR plus intravenous FUDR compared with hepatic arterial FUDR alone has failed to demonstrate any survival advantage for the addition of this systemic approach to regional drug delivery in patients with hepatic metastases from colorectal cancer (Safi et al., 1989).

Two additional points regarding hepatic arterial therapy for colon carcinoma metastatic to the liver are worthy of comment. Because only 40 to 50 percent of patients will be expected to respond to hepatic arterial FUDR, it is important to attempt to identify those patients most likely to respond or, conversely, those individuals who will not benefit from this therapeutic approach. Technetium-99 macroaggregated albumin scans have been used to assist in the positioning of hepatic arterial catheters for the delivery of chemotherapy (Ensminger et al., 1981; Savolaine et al., 1989). In a study reported from the Memorial Sloan-Kettering Cancer Center, 45 percent of patients with good perfusion to the area of tumor demonstrated by the performance of this scan achieved a partial response to treatment compared with only a 13 percent response rate in individuals with poor perfusion ($p = 0.006$) (Kemeny, Niedzwiecki, et al., 1989). Similar results have been reported by investigators at the Dana Farber Institute (Kaplan et al., 1980). Thus, this relatively simple procedure can be used to help select patients who might benefit from hepatic arterial treatment. Unfortunately, it is necessary for the patient to undergo catheter placement before the adequacy of tracer distribution can be assessed. Arteriogram findings have been found to be of little predictive value in defining patients who would respond to this treatment program (Daly et al., 1985).

The second point relates to the question of whether patients should be treated with hepatic arterial chemotherapy only after failure of systemic treatment, if regional therapy does not in fact have an impact on overall survival. With this therapeutic strategy patients whose disease progresses outside the liver will be spared the costs and risks associated with surgical catheter placement.

Although this is not an unreasonable therapeutic approach, it denies the patient with metastatic disease confined to the liver the opportunity to receive treatment that produces the highest objective response rate (with less systemic toxicity). In addition, it is possible that if and when the disease ultimately progresses in the liver the patient may be too ill to undergo a laparotomy catheter insertion. Such patients may be treated by percutaneous catheter placement to deliver the cytotoxic drugs, but this method of treatment is associated with a greater risk of side effects (catheter dislodgement and arterial thrombosis) (Huberman, 1983; Niederhuber and Ensminger, 1983).

Ultimately, it seems most appropriate that the decision about whether and when an individual with colon carcinoma metastatic to the liver should receive hepatic arterial chemotherapy will have to be made based on the unique clinical characteristics of the patient and his or her desire to be treated with this more invasive palliative therapeutic approach (Exhibit 2.3).

3   Intra-arterial Therapy for
       Tumors outside the Liver

3.1 Principles of intra-arterial antineoplastic drug administration

Several basic principles both support and limit the use of intra-arterial anti-neoplastic drug delivery as therapy for tumors outside the liver.

First, as with all forms of regional drug delivery, it is argued that higher doses of a drug in direct contact with a tumor may be translated into an increased response rate and improved survival (Frei and Canellos, 1980; R. O. Stephens, 1988). However, this can only be true if antineoplastic agents active against the tumor are used and there exists a relatively steep dose–response effect for the drug against the malignancy (Frei and Canellos, 1980). In addition, it has been argued that, following local therapy (surgery or radiation therapy), the blood supply to the tumor will be impaired and intra-arterial treatment prior to local therapy (neoadjuvant) will optimize the opportunity to observe the maximal cytotoxic effect (Stephens, 1983).

Second, if intra-arterial therapy is employed with the specific goal of prolonging survival, such an approach should be limited to those clinical situations in which local–regional disease is the major early feature of the tumor and dissemination is known to occur relatively late in the natural history of the malignancy (Stephens, 1983). Treating locally when the tumor has already metastasized widely has little if any chance of affecting the ul-timate outcome. However, if the principal aim of treatment is to palliate local symptoms or to reduce local tumor size prior to surgery or radiation therapy, the "therapeutic benefit" of treatment will be measured differently (i.e., local–regional disease control and extent and duration of pain relief).

Third, it is critical when considering the intra-arterial route of drug deliv-ery to treat only tumors whose nutrient blood supply can be clearly defined to be derived from the artery to be perfused (Szabo et al., 1989). In addition, tumors (e.g., extremity melanomas or sarcomas, head and neck cancers, and brain tumors), supplied by vessels that are easily accessible for catheter placement are the most appropriate candidates for regional vascular drug delivery.

The selection of drugs for intra-arterial administration will depend on the precise therapeutic approach employed. With short-term infusional treatment it will be important to select drugs that are less cell cycle dependent (i.e., alkylating agents and cisplatin). However, if long-term infusions are used, it is reasonable to consider the use of agents such as 5-FU or FUDR, which are active against cycling cells (Chabner et al., 1975).

The major difference between intra-arterial treatment of tumor in the liver and direct vascular drug infusions to other body regions is the relatively limited pharmacokinetic advantage associated with this therapeutic approach in the absence of drug removal (metabolism) prior to its entry into the systemic compartment. However, as noted in Chapter 1, if blood flow through the perfused organ is sluggish and clearance of the drug from the systemic compartment is rapid, a reasonable pharmacokinetic advantage for regional drug delivery may be observed.

In an effort to overcome this potentially serious limitation of regional antineoplastic drug delivery, researchers at a number of centers have explored both experimentally and clinically the technique of *regional isolation/perfusion* (Briele et al., 1985; Oldfield et al., 1985; R. O. Stephens, 1988; Turner et al., 1962). As the name implies, the goal of this treatment program is to isolate both the arterial and venous blood supply to the treated region so that high concentrations of the antineoplastic agent can be perfused (and reperfused) through the tumor-bearing area and then be partially or totally removed before normal circulation is reestablished. Isolation/perfusion technology has its greatest theoretical potential in the treatment of tumors involving the extremities. This technique may allow for a significant increase in short-term tumor exposure to cytotoxic agents while minimizing systemic drug toxicity (Kar et al., 1986). Although the procedure can be repeated more than once, the length of perfusion will be limited by the need to fairly rapidly reestablish the normal blood supply to the body region being perfused.

3.2 Techniques and toxicity of intra-arterial drug delivery

The surgery required to deliver antineoplastic agents by the intra-arterial route will vary considerably with the body region to be perfused and the specific techniques to be employed (e.g., isolation–perfusion) (Krementz, 1986). Major changes in surgical approaches and catheter technology have

Exhibit 3.1
Toxicities of Specific Intra-arterial Treatment Programs

Brain

Eye pain, decreased vision, and blindness (DeWys and Fowler, 1973; Yamada et al., 1979; Stewart, Wallace, et al., 1982; Feun, Wallace, Stewart, et al., 1984; Feun, Wallace, Young, et al., 1984; Feun et al., 1986; Greenberg et al., 1981; Walker et al., 1988)

Seizures (Feun, Wallace, Stewart, et al., 1984; Feun, Wallace, Young, et al., 1984; Feun et al., 1986; Yamada et al., 1979; Madajewicz, West, et al., 1981; Walker et al., 1988)

Hemiparesis (Feun, Wallace, Stewart, et al., 1984; Feun, Wallace, Young, et al., 1984; Feun et al., 1986)

Decreased hearing (Stewart, Wallace, et al., 1982; Mahaley et al., 1989)

Confusion (Yamada et al., 1979; Madajewicz, West, et al., 1981; Walker et al., 1988)

Head and Neck

Decreased vision (Mortimer et al., 1988)

Hemiparesis (Frustack et al., 1986)

Seventh nerve palsy (Mortimer et al., 1988)

Retrobulbar neuritis (Urba and Forastiere, 1986)

Extremities

Edema (Krementz, 1986)

Nerve and muscle damage (Krementz, 1986; Hoekstra et al., 1989; Shiu et al., 1986; Busse, Aigner, and Wilimzig, 1983; Kahn, Messersmith, and Samuels, 1989)

Thrombophlebitis (Krementz, 1986)

Tissue necrosis (Klaase et al., 1989)

Decreased joint mobility (Van Geel, Van Wijk, and Wieberdink, 1989)

Pelvis

Cellulitis (Heim, Eberwein, and Georgi, 1983; Tseng and Park, 1985)

Enterovaginal fistula (Oberfield, 1983b)

Leg pain and nerve damage (Lathrop and Frates, 1983; Eapen et al., 1989; Stewart, Eapen, et al., 1987; Menashe and Jacobs, 1989) markedly reduced the toxicities associated with this method of drug delivery (Krementz, 1986).

The side effects associated with intra-arterial drug delivery can be divided into two general types: systemic and local. The potential severity of systemic side effects will depend on the drug(s) employed, the dose delivered, and the specific intra-arterial technique used. The most serious concern with regional arterial drug administration is the local toxic effects of this therapeutic approach (Krementz, 1986). Again, both the specific types and potential severity of local toxic effects will vary depending on the vessel(s) perfused, the drugs and technique used, and the experience of the team treating the patient.

Side effects common to all forms of intra-arterial therapy include catheter thrombosis, tissue ischemia, bleeding, and infection (Goldman et al., 1975; Krementz, 1986). Toxicities unique to the specific arterial system perfused are listed in Exhibit 3.1.

3.3 Difficulties in assessing the results of intra-arterial therapy for malignant disease

Despite more than 30 years' experience with intra-arterial drug delivery (Sullivan et al., 1953, 1962), the oncology community continues to be uncertain as to what role this therapeutic approach should play in the standard management of individuals with malignant disease. Several explanations can be offered for this state of affairs.

First, the vast majority of reported trials of intra-arterial therapy have been nonrandomized single institutional experiences of highly selected (generally good performance status) patients. This is quite appropriate for an experimental procedure that is associated with the potential for serious morbidity. However, comparing the therapeutic results (survival and palliation) of patients treated in this manner with a historical control population will likely be biased in favor of the aggressively treated patients. This point is of particular significance when survival is the end point being analyzed.

Second, particularly in the older reports of intra-arterial therapy for malignant disease, response criteria were poorly defined, making comparisons with alternative therapeutic strategies quite difficult. This was, and continues to be, a major problem when subjective assessments of effectiveness, such as pain relief, are considered as end points for clinical benefit.

Finally, when objective responses (rather than survival) are used as a measure of clinical utility, careful consideration must be given to the morbidity of the treatment required to obtain tumor shrinkage relative to alternative treatment strategies (i.e., systemic chemotherapy, surgery, and radiation therapy). As noted in Exhibit 3.1, the morbidity of intra-arterial therapy can be considerable. Reports in the medical literature have often failed to critically evaluate this important point. A moderate improvement in a reported response rate for a particular tumor type may not justify acceptance of a therapeutic strategy as standard therapy when the cost, morbidity, and alternative strategies are included in an overall cost-effectiveness analysis. (See Chapter 7 for additional discussion of this issue.)

3.4 Clinical trials of intra-arterial therapy for malignant disease in sites other than the liver

In the following five sections the results of intra-arterial therapy for head and neck cancers, primary and metastatic brain tumors, pelvic tumors, sarcomas, and melanomas of the extremities are briefly reviewed. These are the major tumor types and specific body regions where this therapeutic approach has been attempted and reported in the medical literature.

Unfortunately, as noted in the previous section, even with considerable clinical experience it is often difficult to state definitively under what conditions intra-arterial drug delivery should be considered appropriate standard therapy. However, in the following sections an effort is made to suggest where regional vascular therapy may be reasonably included in the oncologist's management plan and where the approach remains investigational (Exhibit 3.2).

Additional areas where regional arterial drug delivery has been examined include primary lung cancer and metastatic tumors in the lung (Muller, Walther, and Aigner, 1988), gastric cancer (F. O. Stephens, 1988), breast cancer (Aigner et al., 1988; Carter et al., 1988; DeDycker et al., 1988; Koyama et al., 1985; Noguchi et al., 1988; Stephens, 1989), basal cell carcinoma (Chawla et al., 1989), and lymphomas (Jansen et al., 1989). Clinical experience with intra-arterial antineoplastic drug delivery as therapy for these tumor types is too limited to make any statement concerning efficacy relative to other therapeutic options, particularly regarding survival.

However, several series have reported impressive short-term objective response rates following regional vascular drug delivery to the site of local tumor involvement. Of particular interest are recent reports suggesting that as many as 90 percent of patients with locally advanced inoperable breast cancer can be made operable following the use of regional intra-arterial chemotherapy (Carter et al., 1988; DeDycker et al., 1988).

Exhibit 3.2

Current Status of Intra-arterial Therapy (Other Than Hepatic Artery) as Standard Management of Malignant Disease

Proven merit in appropriately selected patients

Advanced local or recurrent melanoma of the extremities

Remains an investigative approach

Adjuvant therapy for melanoma of the extremities

Head and neck cancers

Primary or metastatic brain tumors

Pelvic tumors (gynecologic or gastrointestinal origin)

Sarcomas of the extremities

Other tumor types

3.4.1 Head and neck cancers

There is a large medical literature concerning regional therapy for head and neck cancers that began more than 25 years ago (Baker and Wheeler, 1984; Freckman, 1972; Sullivan et al., 1962).

Several points can be made in support of this approach to the management of this group of malignancies. First, the tumors usually remain confined locally during the early portion of their natural history (Probert, Thompson, and Bagshaw, 1974). Second, a number of antineoplastic agents that may be administered by the intra-arterial route have been demonstrated to have activity in head and neck cancers, including methotrexate and cisplatin (Hong and Bromer, 1983). Third, the vascular supply to the tumors can be easily identified and accessed for direct intra-arterial drug delivery (Baker et al., 1984). Fourth, several experimental models have been developed that provide support for regional drug delivery in this clinical setting (Schouwenburg, Van Putten, and Snow, 1980; Sindram, Snow, and Van Putten, 1974). Finally, limited pharmacokinetic data comparing regional versus intravenous drug administration, as well as actual tumor tissue drug measurements, suggest that higher concentrations of the antineoplastic agents may be reaching the cancer following regional vascular delivery (Gouyette et al., 1986; Wheeler et al., 1986).

Response rates to intra-arterial therapy of 50 to 95 percent have been reported in patients with head and neck cancers previously untreated with chemotherapeutic agents (Baker and Wheeler, 1984; Cheung et al., 1988; Forastiere et al., 1987; Frustaci et al., 1986; Milazzo et al., 1985; Mortimer et al., 1988; Sheen, 1988; Sulfaro et al., 1989). Although these data are impressive, the overall activity observed is similar to that reported with combination systemically delivered chemotherapeutic regimens in head and neck cancer patients who have previously not received chemotherapy or local radiation, or have undergone extensive surgery (Baker and Wheeler, 1984; Hong and Bromer, 1983).

Older trials, including one small randomized clinical trial that suggested a benefit for regional drug delivery compared with local therapy only (Nervi et al., 1978), have often not controlled for the known important prognostic factors in this group of diseases. In addition, the anticipated outcome of adequately staged patients treated in the 1980s with current techniques is frequently superior to that reported in studies of regional drug delivery (Head and Neck Contracts Program, 1987). Also, at least for cisplatin, there is little or no support for an increase in tumor cell kill of head and neck cancer when the dosage of the agent is escalated during systemic drug delivery (Veronesi et al., 1985). Finally, despite high response rates to intra-arterial therapy, disease progression is frequently observed outside the perfused region (Forastiere et al., 1987).

In the absence of large-scale prospective randomized controlled clinical trials it is extremely difficult to compare the results of the regional approach versus systemic chemotherapy administration, because patients treated by the intra-arterial route are likely to be a select group of individuals who the investigators believed would be able to tolerate this difficult and potentially morbid therapeutic program (Carter, 1977). Of note, the use of implantable delivery devices appears to have reduced the toxicity associated with percutaneous intra-arterial infusions and improved patient acceptance of the procedure (Baker and Wheeler, 1982; Baker et al., 1981; Wheeler, Baker, and Medvec, 1984). However, for the present, intra-arterial chemotherapy for head and neck cancers must continue to be regarded as an interesting investigative approach whose eventual role in standard patient management remains to be defined (Baker and Wheeler, 1984).

3.4.2 Primary and metastatic brain tumors

Intracarotid artery antineoplastic drug delivery, principally with cisplatin (40 to 100 mg/m^2) or BCNU (60 to 200 mg/m^2), has been examined for use against both primary and metastatic tumors in the brain (Cascino et al.,

1983; Feun et al., 1986; Feun, Wallace, Stewart, et al., 1984; Feun, Wallace, Yung, et al., 1984; Greenberg et al., 1981; Hidalgo, Hidalgo, and Calvo, 1987; Krementz, 1986; Lehane et al., 1983; Madajewicz, West, et al., 1981; Mahaley et al., 1989; Stewart, Leavens, et al., 1982; Stewart, Wallace, et al., 1982; Weiden, 1988; Yamada et al., 1979). Recently, intra-arterial mitomycin C has also been used against metastatic disease in the brain (Stewart, Grahovac, et al., 1987). Most of the reported series are small (10 to 30 patients) and patient characteristics (i.e., tumor type, prior treatment history, and drug dosages employed) have been quite heterogeneous.

Therefore, it is difficult to draw any firm conclusions concerning the efficacy of this therapeutic approach. Support for the concept of regional drug delivery in the management of primary or metastatic brain tumors is provided by the clinical observation that a tumor perfused by the high concentrations of the antineoplastic agent may respond to therapy while adjacent areas not being directly perfused will not (Weiden, 1988). In addition, in the experimental setting, cisplatin appears to concentrate in brain tissue to a greater extent after intra-arterial drug delivery than after intravenous administration (Madajewicz, Kanter, et al., 1981; Shani et al., 1989).

However, it remains to be determined if this pharmacokinetic advantage can be translated into clinical benefit for patients with primary and metastatic brain tumors, particularly when consideration is given to the potential morbidity associated with this therapeutic approach (Exhibit 3.1). Of note, the preliminary results of a multicenter study comparing intravenous with intra-arterial BCNU in malignant gliomas have failed to demonstrate a survival advantage for patients treated with regional drug delivery (Shapiro et al., 1987). Finally, it must be remembered that whole-brain radiation, the alternative standard treatment of metastatic disease in the brain, frequently results in effective short-term palliation of symptoms with limited morbidity.

3.4.3 Pelvic tumors

Tumors involving the pelvis, including advanced bladder cancer, colorectal cancer, and cancer of the cervix, frequently cause considerable local morbidity. Therefore, regional drug administration can be viewed either as a method of improving survival for this group of diseases or as a technique for treating local symptoms, particularly pain (Oberfield, 1983b).

In the case of advanced bladder cancer, intra-arterial cisplatin plus external radiation has been demonstrated to produce a high objective response rate while avoiding the need for a cystectomy. In one report, 23 of 24 patients (96 percent) treated in this manner achieved a clinical complete response (Eapen et al., 1989). The projected actuarial 2-year survival in this population was 90 percent. Objective response rates of greater than 60 percent have been observed in patients with advanced bladder cancer treated with intra-arterial cisplatin without radiation therapy (Jacobs et al., 1984, 1989; Maatman et al., 1986; Stewart, Eapen, et al., 1987; Stewart et al., 1984; Wallace et al., 1982). Intra-arterial cisplatin has been used at doses ranging from 50 to 150 mg/m^2. It remains to be determined, however, if the response rates observed following treatment with intra-arterial cisplatin are superior to those achieved with intravenous cisplatin-based combination regimens (Yagoda, 1987).

Intra-arterial therapy has also been employed in patients with recurrent colorectal cancer and advanced carcinoma of the cervix. Although occasionally employed as part of the initial treatment program (Rettenmaier et al., 1988), this strategy has most frequently been used to control local symptoms (principally pain) caused by recurrent tumor in the pelvis (Hafstrom et al., 1979; Lathrop and Frates, 1980; Muller, Aigner, and Walther, 1989; O'Keeffe et al., 1989; Swenerton et al., 1979; Tseng and Park, 1985). In one report of patients with colorectal carcinoma treated with intra-arterial mitomycin C (20 mg/m^2), 14 of 30 patients achieved good pain relief despite the fact that only 3 of the 26 evaluable patients demonstrated an objective antitumor response to the treatment program (Tseng and Park, 1985).

3.4.4 Sarcomas

Intra-arterial chemotherapy has been examined in several series of patients with soft tissue sarcomas and osteosarcomas of the extremities. The major justification for this therapeutic approach has been the desire to achieve maximal local tumor cell kill and avoid the need for amputation (Benjamin, 1989; Lawrence, 1988; Stehlin et al., 1975). It has also been hoped that the number of patients eligible for this conservative approach will be increased by using direct intra-arterial therapy to shrink tumor bulk prior to definitive local therapy (i.e., surgery or radiation therapy). An additional goal of preoperative regional vascular drug delivery has been to decrease the risk of spreading viable tumor cells during surgical manipulation of the malignancy (Azzarelli et al., 1983). The major concern with limb-sparing procedures has been that local disease control will be sacrificed and there will be a greater risk for the development of distant metastases.

A number of drugs with at least modest activity in sarcomas, including methotrexate, doxorubicin, and cisplatin, can be considered for intra-arterial therapy in this group of malignancies (Kane, 1989). The earliest trials of adjuvant intra-arterial chemotherapy of sarcomas employed melphalan

(Hoekstra et al., 1987; Lehti et al., 1986; Muchmore, Carter, and Krementz, 1985; Stehlin, 1969). However, more recent investigative efforts involving intra-arterial treatment of sarcomas of the extremities have focused on the use of doxorubicin (40 to 75 mg/m^2) (Eilber, Grant, and Morten, 1978; Eilber et al., 1980, 1984; Jaffe et al., 1978), cisplatin (75 to 150 mg/m^2) (Calvo et al., 1980; Jaffe, Knapp, et al., 1983; Jaffe et al., 1989; Mavligit et al., 1981; Stine et al., 1989); or a combination of the two agents (Stephens et al., 1987).

Substantial tumor necrosis, including complete absence of a viable tumor, has been observed in the tissue specimen obtained at the time of local tumor removal following intra-arterial chemotherapy (Eilber, Grant, and Morten, 1978; Jaffee et al., 1989). In addition, major tumor regression following intra-arterial chemotherapy has been demonstrated on both bone radiographs and angiography (Chuang et al., 1982).

In one of the largest reported series of preoperative intra-arterial chemotherapy (using doxorubicin) for soft tissue sarcomas, 5 of 183 patients (2.7 percent) developed a local recurrence following the completion of the limb-sparing therapeutic protocol (Eilber et al., 1984). Of importance, there was no evidence of a higher systemic relapse rate or lower survival in patients treated with this program compared with a nonrandomized control population who underwent amputation (with adjuvant therapy). However, it remains unknown if patients undergoing a limb-sparing procedure would have done as well with systemic chemotherapy as with intra-arterial drug delivery. This is not a trivial point because the toxicity of intra-arterial doxorubicin can be substantial, including tissue necrosis requiring eventual amputation (Eilber et al., 1984; Klaase et al., 1989).

The local toxicity associated with the intra-arterial delivery of doxorubicin is perhaps the major justification for examining intra-arterial cisplatin in this clinical setting, because the latter agent appears to produce significantly less local toxicity following regional vascular delivery into the extremities (Jaffe et al., 1985). In addition, systemic exposure to cisplatin is not compromised following intra-arterial drug administration (Stewart et al., 1983).

Of interest, although intra-arterial methotrexate did not appear to improve the response rate (approximately 45 percent) for treatment of patients with osteosarcoma of the extremities compared with high-dose intravenous methotrexate (Jaffe, Prudich, et al., 1983), in a small randomized trial comparing intra-arterial cisplatin with high-dose methotrexate, 9 of 15 (60 percent) responded to the regional therapy compared with only 4 of 15 (27 percent) treated systemically (Jaffe et al., 1985). There were 7 complete responses in the cisplatin group and 3 in the methotrexate group. Finally, 2 patients initially treated with intravenous methotrexate who failed this program subsequently received intra-arterial cisplatin and responded.

These initial results are encouraging, but it has yet to be convincingly demonstrated that regional antineoplastic drug delivery results in a survival benefit compared with systemic drug administration (Lawrence, 1988). In addition, the question of whether similar success with limb-sparing procedures can be achieved with intensive combination intravenous chemotherapy remains unanswered (Jaffe et al., 1989). Therefore, for the present, intra-arterial treatment of soft tissue sarcomas and osteosarcoma must be considered a promising experimental therapeutic approach.

3.4.5 Melanomas of the extremities

There is perhaps no more controversial question in oncology than the role of isolation/perfusion therapy in the management of melanomas of the extremities (Cumberlin et al., 1985). A number of recent reviews have critically analyzed the issues involved in this complex subject (Creagan, 1989; Cumberlin et al., 1985; Kroon, 1988; Lee, 1988; Muchmore, Carter, and Krementz, 1985; Voigt, 1988).

Fortunately, there is currently little debate about whether intra-arterial therapy is of clinical benefit for patients with advanced unresectable melanoma, extensive local recurrence, or in-transit metastases. Major palliation can be achieved in 50 to 90 percent of patients treated with regional isolation/perfusion in this clinical setting (Cumberlin et al., 1985; Krementz, 1983; Kroon, 1988; Shiu et al., 1986; Storm and Morton, 1985). In addition, several reports have noted long-term survival in a subset of such patients treated with regional drug delivery (Baas et al., 1988; Shiu et al., 1986).

A number of chemotherapeutic agents have been used for isolation/perfusion of melanomas of the extremities, including nitrogen mustard (Shiu et al., 1986), melphalen (Baas et al., 1989; DiFilippo et al., 1989; Koops and Oldhoff, 1983; Martijn, Oldhoff, and Koops, 1981; Rege et al., 1983; Stehlin, 1969), dacarbazine (Aigner, 1983), and cisplatin (Bland et al., 1989; Calvo et al., 1980; Coit et al., 1989; Pritchard, Mavligit, Benjamin, et al., 1979; Pritchard, Mavligit, Wallace, et al., 1979).

Regional hyperthermia has been used extensively in association with isolation/perfusion of melanomas of the extremities. A number of investigators have suggested that the activity of several chemotherapeutic agents can be enhanced in a hyperthermic environment (Dietzel, 1983; Giovanella, Stehlin, and Morgan, 1976). Unfortunately, no randomized trials comparing hyperthermic with normothermic perfusions have been conducted in the treatment of melanomas of the extremities. However, with few exceptions (Koops et al., 1981; Kroon et al., 1987), most investigators have concluded that the results of isolation/perfusion therapy (response rate and survival) are superior when a hyperthermic (approximately 40 to 42° C) environment is maintained during the perfusion (Cumberlin et al., 1985; DiFilippo et al., 1989; Martijn, Oldhoff, and Koops, 1981; Shiu et al., 1986).

One of the concerns about regional therapy for extremity melanomas has been for any functional impairment that may result from this therapeutic strategy. This issue has been examined by several investigators who have concluded that, in general, patients maintain good function of the treated extremity (Shiu et al., 1986; Van Geel, Van Wijk, and Wieberdink, 1989). Occasionally, patients exhibit decreased joint mobility, atrophy, or edema. The ankle appears to be the joint most severely affected by regional vascular antineoplastic drug delivery (Van Geel, Van Wijk, and Wieberdink, 1989).

Most of the controversy involving intra-arterial isolation/perfusion of melanomas of the extremities centers on its role as an adjuvant treatment following removal of the primary lesion (Cumberlin et al., 1985; Kroon, 1988). In several nonrandomized trials from a number of centers, patients treated with isolation/perfusion following removal of the primary tumor appeared to have a superior prognosis compared with historical controls (Cumberlin et al., 1985; Janoff et al., 1982; Lee, 1988a, 1988b; Rege et al., 1983; Sugarbaker and McBride, 1976; Tonak et al., 1983).

A single randomized trial that did suggest a benefit for adjuvant hyperthermic regional therapy in patients with melanomas of the extremities has been criticized for its small sample size (Ghussen et al., 1984, 1988). For example, in this study there were a total of only 18 Stage 1 patients in the control arm and 19 in the perfusion group of this trial.

The difficulty in assessing the value of adjuvant therapy for melanomas of the extremities on the basis of nonrandomized clinical experience is compounded by the known heterogenesis biology of this malignancy and the importance of specific clinical features (including stage and tumor thickness), which are of great prognostic significance (Lee, 1988a, 1988b).

One example of the use of historical control populations to assess the value of regional isolation/perfusion as adjuvant therapy of melanomas of the extremities dramatically illustrates the danger associated with this analytical method. In 1986, a Dutch group reported the results of adjuvant isolation/perfusion of melanomas of the extremities and compared these findings with a carefully matched Australian patient population who had not received adjuvant treatment (Martijn et al., 1986). The report concluded that women (the only group with adequate patient numbers for comparison) treated with intra-arterial melphalan experienced significantly higher 10-year disease-free ($p < 0.0005$) and overall ($p < 0.025$) survivals compared with the untreated nonrandomized control population.

However, when the same analysis was performed using the identical treated population and a matched control group from the Netherlands, there was no difference in either disease-free or overall survival (Franklin et al., 1988). As with many other questions concerning the peculiar biology of melanomas, there is no obvious explanation for why Australian patients with localized melanomas of the extremities have a poorer survival than Dutch patients with what appears to be identical clinical characteristics.

In summary, intra-arterial isolation/perfusion of unresectable, recurrent, or locally metastatic melanomas of the extremities has been shown to be effective in palliating symptoms and producing long-term disease-free survival in a subset of treated patients. Unequivocal clinical benefit for this technique in the adjuvant setting following surgical tumor removal has not been established. It will be only through the conduct of large-scale prospective randomized clinical trials that the role for this therapeutic approach can be established.

It is important to remember that patients with locally advanced or recurrent disease who are candidates for local therapy form a unique subset of individuals with this condition, because their disease will likely not have manifested itself by the development of distant metastases (i.e., lung, liver, and brain). Thus, it is inappropriate to assume that clinical benefit observed in the advanced localized setting can automatically be translated into an effective therapeutic strategy when all patients with early-stage melanomas of the extremities are considered (adjuvant treatment).

4   Intraperitoneal Therapy

4.1 Scope of the clinical issues and alternative treatment options

4.1.1 Ovarian cancer

Approximately twenty thousand new cases of ovarian cancer are discovered in the United States each year, 70 to 80 percent of which will be found to be advanced (Stage III or IV) disease at initial presentation (Silverberg and Lubera, 1989). Even though 60 to 80 percent of patients with ovarian cancer will respond to systemic cisplatin-based chemotherapy (the single most active drug in this disease), less than 25 percent of patients will be alive and disease free more than 5 years after diagnosis (Louie et al., 1986; Ozols and Young, 1987; Silverberg and Lubera, 1989). Perhaps even more discouraging is the recently recognized fact that 50 to 60 percent of women with high-grade ovarian tumors who experience a surgically defined complete response with cisplatin-based chemotherapy will ultimately relapse (Cain et al., 1986; Copeland and Gershenson, 1986; Rubin, Hoskins, Saigo, et al., 1988).

Although responses to second-line chemotherapy may be observed (10 to 20 percent or less of patients treated), such responses are usually of short duration (< 4 to 6 months) (Chambers et al., 1987; Laufman et al., 1986; Pater et al., 1987; Stanhope, Smith, and Rutledge, 1977). Whole-abdominal radiation therapy in refractory ovarian cancer has been advocated by some, but most studies have not demonstrated that this potentially morbid therapeutic approach results in significant prolongation of survival (Fuller et al., 1987; Hoskins et al., 1985; Shelly et al., 1988).

Of particular relevance to the question of the potential clinical utility of intraperitoneal therapy in the management of ovarian cancer is the observation that the tumor remains largely confined to the peritoneal cavity (at least from the perspective of clinical symptoms) for most of its natural history in the majority of individuals afflicted with this disease (Bergman, 1966; Dauplat et al., 1987; Obel, 1976).

4.1.2 Peritoneal mesothelioma

Because most authors have failed to separate the natural history and results of treatment of peritoneal mesothelioma from those of pleural mesothelioma, it is difficult to precisely define the characteristics (i.e., median- and long-term survival and response rate to systemic therapy) of the malignant condition that principally involves the peritoneal cavity (Antman, 1981; Antman et al., 1988; Elmes and Simpson, 1976). Ten to thirty percent of mesotheliomas have been considered to be peritoneal in origin (or at least cause their major morbidity in this region of the body) (Antman, 1981; Plaus, 1988). The median life expectancy for a patient with malignant mesothelioma is approximately 15 months, with few patients living more than 4 years (Antman et al., 1988; Lerner et al., 1983; Plaus, 1988). Although several chemotherapeutic agents have been demonstrated to have limited activity in malignant mesothelioma (Aisner and Wiernik, 1981; Bajorin, Kelsen, and Mintzer, 1987; Chahinian et al., 1984; Mintzer et al., 1985), it has been questioned whether systemic chemotherapy has had any meaningful impact on the natural history of this disease (Alberts et al., 1988; Pisani, Colby, and Williams, 1988).

4.1.3 Gastrointestinal malignancies

The metastatic pattern of gastrointestinal malignancies differs considerably from that of ovarian carcinoma and of peritoneal mesothelioma, with spread to the liver being a major feature of this group of diseases. However, local peritoneal cavity recurrences remain a serious problem for these common malignancies (Douglass, 1985; Silverberg and Lubera, 1989; Sugarbaker et al., 1988).

4.2 Rationale for intraperitoneal therapy for ovarian cancer, peritoneal mesothelioma, and gastrointestinal malignancies

The principal rationale for treating any malignancy by the intraperitoneal route of drug delivery is that a tumor present in the cavity can be exposed to higher concentrations of the drug for longer periods of time than can be accomplished by the systemic administration of the agents. Essential to any argument supporting the superiority of intraperitoneal over systemic drug delivery is the expectation that this increased exposure can be translated into a greater cytotoxic effect (Frei and Canellos, 1980; Samson et al., 1984).

For example, in the case of ovarian cancer clinically refractory to systemic cisplatin, there are both clinical and in vitro data to suggest that the higher concentrations of the agent achievable in the peritoneal cavity following intraperitoneal delivery (10- to 20-fold compared with intravenous administration [Casper et al., 1983; Howell et al., 1982; Lopez et al., 1985]) can overcome the resistance that develops following exposure of the cancer to lower concentrations of the drug (Bruckner et al., 1981; Levin and Hryniuk, 1987; Ozols et al., 1985; Ozols and Young, 1987). In experimental systems it has been difficult to make ovarian cancer cells more than severalfold resistant to cisplatin, an observation that lends support to the concept that intraperitoneal therapy with this agent may play an important role in the management of ovarian cancer (Andrews et al., 1988).

Regarding peritoneal mesothelioma, very limited experimental data are available to support the use of a particular chemotherapeutic agent for regional therapy (Aisner and Wiernik, 1981). The recently demonstrated ability of surgeons to successfully debulk the patient with peritoneal mesothelioma to small residual tumor volumes at least makes it possible to test the concept of intraperitoneal therapy in this disease setting (Antman et al., 1985; Lederman et al., 1987).

The rationale for employing intraperitoneal therapy as treatment for gastrointestinal malignancies has been described in detail by several authors (Markman, 1987b; Speyer, 1985; Sugarbaker et al., 1988). There are several major arguments supporting this approach as part of the management plan of gastrointestinal malignancies.

First, in several tumor types (i.e., gastric and colon cancer) it has been demonstrated that recurrences following "curative" surgical resections frequently involve the peritoneal cavity (Douglass, 1985; Sugarbaker et al., 1988). In addition, in gastric cancer, free-floating viable-appearing tumor cells can be found within the cavity at the time of surgical resection (Iitsuka et al., 1979; Martin and Goellner, 1986; Nakajima et al., 1978).

The extremely high concentrations of the drug achieved within the peritoneal cavity may be capable of killing microscopic disease present at the time of curative surgical resection (adjuvant therapy). Although it is unknown whether local control of disease can be translated into a decrease in systemic recurrences and improved survival, in theory it can at least be argued that spread of disease to the liver and systemic compartment is via the peritoneal cavity and that preventing the growth of cells in the cavity will inhibit further progression of the malignant process.

Second, experimental data have demonstrated that the uptake of drugs the size of most chemotherapeutic agents from the peritoneal cavity is principally via the portal circulation (Kraft, Tompkins, and Jesseph, 1968; Lukas, Brindle, and Greengard, 1971). Microscopic tumor present in the liver and receiving its blood supply from the portal vein may be killed at concentrations of cytotoxic agents (such as 5-FU) achieved in the portal circulation following intraperitoneal administration (see Section 2.2 in Chapter 2 for additional discussion of the rationale for portal vein drug delivery as adjuvant therapy following curative surgery of colon cancer). Again, the overall impact on patient survival, even if this approach is successful in preventing tumor progression in the liver, is uncertain.

Finally, the selection of agents for intraperitoneal delivery that are rapidly and extensively metabolized into nontoxic metabolites during their first passage through the liver allows for an escalation of drug delivery and an increase in exposure of tumor present in the cavity and liver to the cytotoxic drug. This argument assumes that such dose escalations will not produce excessive local toxicity to the peritoneal lining or liver. For 5-FU, the single most important drug in the treatment of gastrointestinal malignancies, there is both a major pharmacokinetic advantage for peritoneal cavity and portal vein exposure and an acceptable toxicity profile for local and systemic side effects when the agent is delivered by the intraperitoneal route (Reichman et al., 1988; Speyer et al., 1980, 1981).

4.3 Technical considerations and practical/theoretical limitations of intraperitoneal therapy

As with regional therapeutic approaches employing the vascular compartment, it is critical that the establishment of a safe and convenient access to the peritoneal cavity be carefully considered. Intermittent percutaneous placement of peritoneal catheters, often performed under ultrasonic or laparoscopic guidance at the time of each treatment, has been employed by investigators experienced with this approach (e.g., Runowicz et al., 1986). Unfortunately, the risk of inadvertent bowel perforation, particularly in individuals without ascites who have undergone one or more previous laparotomies with resultant adhesion formation, is a cause of genuine concern (Kaplan et al., 1985).

Surgical placement of semipermanent indwelling catheters (Tenckhoff type), commonly employed in peritoneal dialysis, has greatly simplified treatment delivery (Jenkins et al., 1982; Piccart et al., 1985). Catheters either can be placed at the time of a planned laparotomy to assess the status of disease (second-look laparotomy) or to debulk tumor, or can be inserted at the time of a more limited procedure performed specifically for that purpose (Lucas, 1984; Rubin, Hoskins, Markman, et al., 1988). The recent availability of totally subcutaneous delivery devices has improved patient acceptance of the presence of the indwelling catheter and appears to have reduced the incidence of catheter infection (Piccart et al., 1985; Pfeifle et al., 1984; Kaplan et al., 1985). However, it must be noted that there continue to be problems associated with the use of these devices, including difficulty with fluid flow through the catheters (particularly outflow), fluid extravasation, bowel perforation, and infection (Braly, Doroshow, and Hoff, 1986; Degraff et al., 1988; Kerr et al., 1987; Markman and Kelsen, 1989; Pfeifle et al., 1985; Piccart et al., 1985; Rubin, Hoskins, Markman, et al., 1988; Varney et al., 1989; Wakefield et al., 1984; Walton, 1989).

In contrast to those situations where the vascular compartment is employed in regional therapy to deliver the drug to the tumor, it cannot be assumed that high concentrations of the cytotoxic agent will reach the site of the malignancy simply by administering the drug into the peritoneal cavity. It has clearly been demonstrated both experimentally and by clinical experience that when small volumes of fluid are employed to instill a drug into the peritoneal cavity, distribution of the agent throughout the cavity is unsatisfactory (Rosenshein et al., 1978; Taylor et al., 1985; Vider, Deland, and Maruyama, 1976). This is particularly true in patients who have significant adhesion formation from previous abdominal surgeries.

Fortunately, several small trials have suggested that if relatively large treatment volumes are employed (at least 2 l), distribution of drug-containing fluid is adequate to bathe the entire peritoneal cavity (as determined by radiographic evaluation) in the majority of patients considered for this treatment approach (Dunnick et al., 1979; Howell et al., 1982; Levenback et al., 1989). Methods of assessing drug distribution include either a computerized tomographic scan with intraperitoneal contrast or a nuclear medicine scan with intraperitoneally administered radiolabeled material (Dunnick et al., 1979; Howell et al., 1982; Levenback et al., 1989; Van Weelde et al., 1984).

There continues to be concern that even if the initial distribution appears to be adequate (by radiologic assessment) for intraperitoneal treatment, there will be clinical or subclinical inflammation associated with the therapy leading to additional adhesion formation and worsening of drug distribution with subsequent treatments. The severity of this problem will likely vary considerably based on the sclerosing potential of the drug(s) employed. A preliminary report from the Memorial Sloan-Kettering Cancer Center examining the distribution of intraperitoneally administered radiolabeled albumin over the course of intraperitoneal treatment has suggested that although changes are observed in many individuals during the course of their therapy, severe maldistribution is uncommon in patients who initially demonstrate good intraperitoneal distribution of the tracer (Levenback et al., in press).

There are two additional and related issues that critics of the intraperitoneal approach to the management of malignant disease appropriately note and that significantly limit those clinical situations where intraperitoneal therapy can be considered a reasonable therapeutic option. These are (a) the concern that intraperitoneal therapy will decrease the delivery of the cytotoxic drug to the tumor by capillary flow and (b) the limited penetration of the drug into the tumor by free-surface diffusion.

When a chemotherapeutic agent is administered intravenously it reaches the tumor by capillary flow. A variable portion of a drug administered intraperitoneally will also be delivered to the tumor via this mechanism, depending on the amount of the active drug that exits the cavity and enters the systemic compartment. Systemic exposure will be limited (compared with cavity exposure) following intraperitoneal delivery for drugs that are extensively metabolized into nontoxic metabolites during their first passage through the liver (i.e., 5-FU and cytarabine) or for drugs that are deposited in tissue and never leave the body cavity (i.e., mitoxantrone) (Alberts et al., 1985; Chabner et al., 1975; Savaraj et al., 1982).

Conversely, systemic exposure to agents that undergo minimal inactivation following intraperitoneal delivery will be substantial and may equal that achieved with systemic drug delivery (i.e., cisplatin and carboplatin). The issue that arises from these considerations relates to the concern that although local tumor–drug interactions may be enhanced following intraperitoneal administration, systemic exposure to the drug and delivery to the site of the malignancy may be compromised, resulting in an overall decrease in therapeutic efficacy.

The selection of agents for intraperitoneal administration that ultimately reach the tumor by capillary flow in an active form at the same concentration as if they were delivered by the systemic route should minimize this concern (Litterst, Torres, et al., 1982). Alternatively, one could administer an individual drug both intravenously and by the intraperitoneal route, or deliver a second drug intravenously (e.g., cisplatin) along with an agent instilled intraperitoneally that is known to essentially have only a local effect (e.g., mitoxantrone).

The final issue of concern relates to the known limited direct penetration of chemotherapeutic agents into both normal and tumor tissue (delivery by free-surface diffusion). In a number of experimental systems examining several chemotherapeutic agents, including doxorubicin (Durand, 1981; Ozols, Locker, Doroshow, et al., 1979b); methotrexate (West, Weichselbau, and Little, 1980), 5-FU (Nederman and Carlsson, 1984), and cisplatin (Los et al., 1989), the direct penetration into tissue has been found to range from a minimum of 4 to 6 cell layers to a maximum of several millimeters.

Of considerable interest and importance to the issue of the penetration of chemotherapeutic agents is the recent work from the Netherlands Cancer Center, where the penetration of cisplatin into tumor tissue in a rat tumor model was examined (Los et al., 1989). This group found that although cisplatin could be measured in tumor tissue to a depth exceeding 2 mm from the peritoneal surface, the advantage associated with intraperitoneal administration (compared with that of intravenous delivery of the drug) was confined to a depth of only 1 mm from the peritoneal surface.

This work, as well as experimental and clinical data provided by other investigators, would strongly suggest that any advantage of intraperitoneal therapy over systemic drug delivery will be limited to those clinical situations where only microscopic disease or very small tumor nodules (0.5 cm or less) are present when intraperitoneal treatment is initiated. These data also provide important support for the concept of extensive surgical debulking of intraperitoneal disease, if necessary, prior to the initiation of intraperitoneal therapy (Heintz et al., 1986; Piver and Baker, 1986; Silberman, 1982). Such surgery will enable intraperitoneal drug delivery to have a realistic opportunity to favorably affect the ultimate outcome of the underlying disease process.

4.4 Early clinical experience with intracavitary treatment and the intracavitary use of antineoplastic agents for their sclerosing rather than cytotoxic properties

In the early days of the modern chemotherapeutic era (1950–1970), clinical researchers administered a number of agents by the intraperitoneal route, including nitrogen mustard (Weisberger, Levine, and Storaasli, 1955), hemisulfur mustard (Green, 1959), thiotepa (Kottmeier, 1968), and 5-FU (Clarkson, 1964; Clarkson et al., 1964; Suhrland and Weisberger, 1965). Although "clinical responses" were observed (reduction in ascites accumulation and improvement in "quality of life"), there was little evidence that the drugs were doing more than causing sclerosis of the cavity and mechanically preventing fluid reaccumulation. In addition, toxicity (principally abdominal pain) was occasionally severe and bulky tumor masses rarely, if ever, responded to such treatment. Therefore, it is not surprising that there was little enthusiasm in the oncology community for the intraperitoneal delivery of antineoplastic drugs for the purpose of producing a cytotoxic rather than a sclerosing effect.

Several antineoplastic agents have been extensively investigated for intracavitary administration specifically to prevent the reaccumulation of malignant effusions. These include nitrogen mustard (Austin and Flye, 1979), bleomycin (Bitran et al., 1981; Ostrowski, 1986; Ostrowski and Halsall, 1982; Paladine et al., 1976), and doxorubicin (Kefford et al., 1980). There is also more limited experience employing cisplatin for both intrapleural (Markman, Howell, and Green, 1984; Markman et al., 1985), and intrapericardial administration (Fiorentino et al., 1988; Markman and Howell, 1985b) in the management of malignant effusions.

Although major clinical benefit has been noted when using these agents (particularly bleomycin), it remains unclear whether there is any advantage of using such drugs over agents that appear to be equally effective in producing a sclerosing effect (e.g., tetracycline and talc) but are not associated with systemic side effects (Austin and Flye, 1979; Davis, Rambotti, and Grignani, 1984; Fentiman, 1987; Hausheer and Yarbro, 1984).

It is important to remember in the following discussion of the potential efficacy of the intraperitoneal use of antineoplastic agents that success in controlling malignant ascites with certain drugs may be at least partially explained by cavity sclerosis rather than a direct cytotoxic effect.

4.5 Phase 1 trials of intraperitoneal therapy

There were several reasons why, in the late 1970s, interest in the intraperitoneal administration of chemotherapeutic agents was renewed. First, a number of new highly active drugs that had not previously been delivered by the intraperitoneal route, including cisplatin, were introduced into clinical practice. Second, safe methods for regional drug delivery, including the Tenckhoff catheter, were developed (Twardowski, 1985). Finally, investigators at the National Cancer Institute, using known anatomic and physiologic characteristics of the peritoneal cavity and pharmacologic properties of the available chemotherapeutic agents, developed a mathematical model that strongly suggested there should be a significant increase in exposure of

Table 4.1

Pharmacokinetic Advantage of Intraperitoneal Drug Delivery

| Drug | Mean peritoneal cavity/plasma concentration ratio | |
	Peak levels	AUC[a]
Methotrexate	92	—
5-Fluorouracil	298	367
Fluorodeoxyuridine	—	1,000
Cisplatin	20	12
Carboplatin	—	18
Doxorubicin	474	—
Mitoxantrone	—	1,400
Melphalan	93	65
Thiotepa	—	4
Mitomycin C	71	—
Cytarabine	664	474
Streptozocin	40	—
Etoposide	—	65[b]

[a] Area-under-concentration-versus-time curve.
[b] Non-protein-bound drug.

the peritoneal cavity to certain drugs (compared with the systemic circulation) when the agents were instilled directly into the cavity (Dedrick, 1985; Dedrick et al., 1978).

These factors led to the conduct of a number of Phase 1 single-agent intraperitoneal trials, the results of which are briefly summarized below (also see Table 4.1).

4.5.1 Methotrexate

There are several reasons why methotrexate was one of the first drugs to be examined for intraperitoneal administration. First, the drug is known to have activity in ovarian cancer (Thigpen et al., 1987). Second, because methotrexate had previously been administered intrathecally in the treatment of meningeal leukemia (see Chapter 6), it was felt the drug would not produce excessive local toxicity when delivered by the intraperitoneal route. Finally, methotrexate has a known antidote (leucovorin) that can prevent toxicity produced by the cytotoxic drug (Chabner et al., 1975). Several investigators suggested that it might be possible to significantly increase both the total dose of methotrexate delivered by the intraperitoneal route and the length of exposure of tumor present within the cavity to this antimetabolite by administering leucovorin systemically with intraperitoneal methotrexate delivery (Howell et al., 1981; Jones et al., 1981).

A major pharmacokinetic advantage for the intraperitoneal administration of methotrexate was demonstrated in these trials (Table 4.1) when systemic leucovorin was delivered either to neutralize the cytotoxic drug escaping from the cavity during the methotrexate installation (Howell et al., 1981) or to rescue the patient following the completion of the intraperitoneal instillation (Jones et al., 1981). Dose-limiting toxicity was found to be both systemic (principally thrombocytopenia) and local (abdominal pain). In the initial Phase 1 trials clinical responses were observed (principally reduction in ascites formation) in several patients.

Of considerable interest is the recent report from investigators at the Memorial Sloan-Kettering Cancer Center demonstrating that 10-ethyl-10-deazaaminopterin (10-EDAM), a compound closely related to methotrexate, is markedly synergistic with cisplatin when administered intraperitoneally as treatment of a human ovarian carcinoma cell line growing intraperitoneally (Sirotnak et al., 1989). Conversely, methotrexate plus cisplatin was observed to be only modestly active in this experimental system. Further exploration of this new compound in clinical intraperitoneal trials appears indicated.

4.5.2 Fluorouracil

As previously noted, 5-FU has a long history as an agent used to prevent malignant peritoneal fluid reaccumulation. However, it has only been within the past 10 years that a firm pharmacokinetic basis for the intraperitoneal administration of this drug has been established (Demicheli et al., 1982; Gyves, 1985; Gyves et al., 1984; Speyer et al., 1980). Following the intraperitoneal instillation of 5-FU, the peritoneal cavity demonstrates a 2- to 3-log increased exposure to the agent compared with that of the systemic circulation (Table 4.1). Of particular interest to the question of a role for intraperitoneal 5-FU as adjuvant therapy of gastrointestinal malignancies was the observation by investigators at the National Cancer Institute that portal vein levels of 5-FU following intraperitoneal administration are comparable to hepatic artery levels of the agent following direct hepatic artery infusions (Speyer et al., 1981). This experimental data would suggest that adequate concentrations of 5-FU are achieved in the portal circulation to potentially treat micrometastatic disease present in the liver (Speyer, 1985).

In addition, in one experimental system, the intraperitoneal administration of 5-FU demonstrated comparable pharmacokinetics to portal vein drug delivery (Archer, McCulloch, and Gray, 1989). Of further interest, the "streaming effect" noted with regional vascular drug delivery (see Section 2.2 in Chapter 2) was not observed with intraperitoneal drug administration. In theory this may be an important advantage for intraperitoneal therapy over portal vein drug delivery in the adjuvant setting.

In the several Phase 1 trials of intraperitoneal 5-FU reported, the agent has been administered once daily or on multiple occasions each day by dialysis exchange. Dose-limiting toxicity appears to be both the local and systemic effects of the drug. In general, the acute pain associated with intraperitoneal 5-FU administration is mild in severity (Gianola et al., 1986; Reichman et al., 1988; Speyer et al., 1980). However, the agent can result in subclinical irritation of the peritoneal lining, often leading to significant adhesion formation. Following several courses of treatment more severe abdominal pain may be observed after drug instillation. In patients who have been heavily pretreated with systemic chemotherapy, intraperitoneal 5-FU may result in bone marrow suppression (Reichman et al., 1988). However, in patients previously untreated with chemotherapy, the marrow-suppressive effects of intraperitoneal 5-FU are generally mild (Gianola et al., 1986).

A recently reported Phase 1 trial from the Memorial Sloan-Kettering Cancer Center has examined the simultaneous daily intraperitoneal administration of single-agent 5-FU along with the continuous intravenous infusion of the agent (Reichman et al., 1988). This regimen was designed to take advantage of the high local drug concentrations achieved in the peritoneal cavity following intraperitoneal administration and the continuous exposure of the tumor to this cell-cycle-specific drug (Chabner et al., 1975). A 4-day regimen of intraperitoneal 5-FU (1,000 mg/day) and intravenous 5-FU (1,000 mg/m^2/day) was found to be reasonably well tolerated. In this and other Phase 1 trials of intraperitoneal 5-FU, limited activity has been demonstrated in gastrointestinal malignancies and refractory ovarian cancer.

Intraperitoneal 5-FU has also been examined in a small trial as adjuvant treatment following resection of hepatic metastases from colorectal cancer (August et al., 1985). Although the program was well tolerated, there was no evidence that the adjuvant treatment improved survival compared with a nonrandomized population treated with surgery alone. This approach has also been applied in a small number of patients with unresectable metastases from colorectal cancer, with marginal evidence of therapeutic benefit (Ekberg et al., 1988).

4.5.3 Fluorodeoxyuridine

Although there is far less experience with the intraperitoneal delivery of FUDR than with 5-FU, for the reasons discussed in Section 2.5 in Chapter 2, there has been considerable recent interest in examining the safety, pharmacokinetics, and potential clinical efficacy of FUDR following intraperitoneal administration (Muggia et al., 1988; Smith et al., 1989). As might have been anticipated from knowledge of the pharmacokinetics of hepatic arterial infusions of 5-FU and FUDR, following the intraperitoneal administration of FUDR the advantage for cavity exposure appears to be superior to that observed with 5-FU (Muggia et al., 1988). As with 5-FU, dose-limiting toxicity is both local (abdominal pain and adhesion formation following several treatment courses) and systemic (diarrhea and marrow suppression in heavily pretreated patients).

At the present time there is limited clinical experience employing single-agent intraperitoneal FUDR, and it is not possible to make any statement regarding its efficacy relative to that of 5-FU. One recommended intraperitoneal FUDR treatment regimen for Phase 2 testing calls for the agent to be administered at a daily dose of 3 to 4 g/day for 3 days, with treatment repeated monthly (Muggia et al., 1988).

4.5.4 Cisplatin

Cisplatin is considered the single most important drug in the treatment of ovarian carcinoma (Ozols and Young, 1987; Thigpen et al., 1987). Therefore, it is not surprising that cisplatin has been the most studied agent for intraperitoneal administration (Lagasse et al., 1981; Sekiya, Iwasawa, and Takamizawa, 1985). Several Phase 1 trials have confirmed a 10- to 20-fold increased exposure for the peritoneal cavity compared with that of the systemic compartment following the intraperitoneal administration of cisplatin (Casper et al., 1983; Esposito et al., 1988; Howell et al., 1982, 1983; Lopez et al., 1985; Pretorius et al., 1983). As previously noted, this modest pharmacokinetic advantage for intraperitoneal delivery is of significant interest because cancer cells from ovarian cancer patients with tumors "clinically resistant" to cisplatin have been found to be only severalfold resistant in vitro to concentrations of the agent achievable in the systemic circulation (Andrews et al., 1988; Ozols, Cordon, et al., 1984).

In a number of Phase 1 trials, intraperitoneal cisplatin has been found to produce clinical responses in patients with refractory ovarian cancer and peritoneal mesothelioma. As suggested by the previous discussion of the penetration of cisplatin into tumor tissue, shrinkage of bulky intra-abdominal disease in patients with refractory ovarian cancer has rarely been observed.

Of great importance, intraperitoneal cisplatin has been found to cause limited local toxicity. Acute abdominal pain is infrequent and when it occurs is often the result of preexisting adhesions from prior surgery. At exploratory laparotomy filmy adhesions are commonly encountered, but intraperitoneal cisplatin-induced bowel obstruction is very uncommon (Markman et al., 1986). It is important to note that cisplatin-based combination intraperitoneal therapy may result in more extensive local irritation, either due solely to the additional drugs included in the regimen or secondary to an adverse interaction between the agents employed (Markman et al., 1984).

The dose-limiting toxicities of intraperitoneal cisplatin are the systemic side effects of the agent, because the majority of the cisplatin infused into the peritoneal cavity will ultimately enter the systemic compartment (Howell et al., 1982; Pretorius et al., 1983). This is an important point to remember because it would be inappropriate to treat a patient with cisplatin by the intraperitoneal route (rather than intravenously) in the hope of preventing emesis or a worsening of a preexisting cisplatin-induced neuropathy or nephropathy.

Investigators at the University of California, San Diego (UCSD), have explored the use of intraperitoneal cisplatin along with systemically delivered sodium thiosulfate used to prevent cisplatin-induced nephrotoxicity (Howell et al., 1982, 1983; Lucas, Markman, and Howell, 1985). Sodium thiosulfate has a long history of safe use in humans as therapy for cyanide poisoning (Chen and Rose, 1952). Previous work from the UCSD group had demonstrated that thiosulfate completely inactivates both the nephrotoxic and cytotoxic properties of cisplatin (Howell and Taetle, 1980). However, it appears that at the relatively low concentrations of thiosulfate present in the plasma or peritoneal cavity very limited amounts of cisplatin are inactivated, while the higher concentration of thiosulfate in the kidney is capable of protecting that organ from serious damage (Shea, Koziol, and Howell, 1984).

In a Phase 1 trial of escalating doses of intraperitoneal cisplatin, the UCSD investigators were able to deliver cisplatin up to a dose of 270 mg/m^2 without producing significant nephrotoxicity (Howell et al., 1982, 1983).

Of note, despite the use of this extremely high level of cisplatin, little local toxicity (pain or adhesion formation) was observed. At the present time it is unknown if the somewhat higher concentrations of cisplatin achieved in the peritoneal cavity following the intraperitoneal delivery of this agent with simultaneous intravenous thiosulfate offers any clinical benefit over that accomplished by a lower intraperitoneal dose of cisplatin (approximately 100 mg/m^2) without thiosulfate. Randomized controlled clinical trials will be required to answer this important question.

4.5.5 Carboplatin and iproplatinum

Carboplatin has been demonstrated in several clinical trials to have a spectrum of activity similar to that of cisplatin, with a significantly different toxicity profile (Muggia, 1989). For this reason there has been considerable interest in the intraperitoneal administration of this agent. The pharmacokinetic advantage associated with intraperitoneal delivery has been shown to be similar to that of cisplatin (Table 4.1) (Colombo et al., 1987; Deregorio et al., 1986; Elferink et al., 1988; McVie et al., 1985). As with cisplatin, local toxicity is minimal. Finally, as would be expected from the known toxicity profile of intravenously delivered drug, dose-limiting toxicity is bone marrow suppression (principally thrombocytopenia).

The pharmacokinetics of intraperitoneally administered iproplatinum have also been examined in a small Phase 1 trial, with a 30-fold increased exposure of the peritoneal cavity compared with the systemic circulation being demonstrated (Kerr et al., 1988).

4.5.6 Doxorubicin

On the basis of an experimental mouse model of ovarian carcinoma in which intraperitoneal doxorubicin was shown to "cure"the malignancy while intravenous therapy with the same agent resulted in death of the animals, considerable enthusiasm was generated for exploring the intraperitoneal use of this agent in patients (Ozols, Grotzinger, et al., 1979; Ozols, Locker, et al., 1979). In addition, doxorubicin is known to have activity in ovarian carcinoma and is one of the drugs commonly employed in cisplatin-based combination therapy programs (Thigpen et al., 1987). In several Phase 1 trials a major pharmacokinetic advantage for peritoneal cavity exposure following intraperitoneal delivery of doxorubicin was demonstrated (Table 4.1) (Demicheli et al., 1985; Ozols et al., 1982).

Unfortunately, and not surprisingly in view of the known vesicant properties of doxorubicin (Litterst, Collins, et al., 1982), local toxicity (abdominal pain and adhesion formation) with intraperitoneal drug administration was found to be substantial (Demicheli et al., 1985; Ozols et al., 1982; Roboz et al., 1981).

Clinical responses to intraperitoneal doxorubicin were noted by several investigators in refractory ovarian cancer. However, with several notable exceptions (Antman et al., 1985; Sugarbaker et al., 1988), most investigators feel this agent is too toxic locally for standard clinical use.

4.5.7 Mitoxantrone

Mitoxantrone, a dihydroxyquinone derivative of anthracene, has been found to have a spectrum of toxicity and clinical activity similar to that of doxorubicin when the two agents are delivered by the intravenous route (Schenkenberg and Von Hoff, 1986). However, for a number of reasons, it was believed appropriate by several groups to examine the intraperitoneal administration of mitoxantrone, despite the previous disappointing experience with doxorubicin.

First, mitoxantrone has been shown to have activity in ovarian cancer when delivered as a single agent by the intravenous route (Lawton et al., 1987). Second, in contrast to doxorubicin, mitoxantrone is not considered to be a vesicant, suggesting it might produce relatively less local toxicity than doxorubicin when administered by the intraperitoneal route (Dorr, Alberts, and Soble, 1986; Schenkenberg and Von Hoff, 1986). Finally, work by investigators at the University of Arizona Cancer Center employing the human tumor stem cell assay suggested that at concentrations of mitoxantrone achievable in the peritoneal cavity following intraperitoneal administration, greater than 90 percent of malignant epithelial ovarian tumors are successfully killed by the agent (Alberts, Young, et al., 1985). These authors noted that mitoxantrone was the single most active commercially available agent they had tested in this in vitro system for potential intraperitoneal administration against ovarian cancer.

Several Phase 1 trials of intraperitoneal mitoxantrone have been reported (Alberts et al., 1988; Blochl-Daum et al., 1987, 1988; Loeffler and Freund, 1986; McVie et al., 1987). A remarkable 1,400-fold increased exposure of the peritoneal cavity to mitoxantrone following intraperitoneal delivery has been observed (Alberts et al., 1988). This striking finding appears to be due to both inactivation of mitoxantrone in the liver and deposition of the drug in tissue (Alberts, Peng, et al., 1985; Savaraj et al., 1982; Stewart et al., 1986). It is likely that a substantial portion of the agent never leaves the peritoneal cavity.

This finding leads to the provocative suggestion that the intraperitoneal administration of mitoxantrone might result in a "depot effect," whereby multiple layers of tumor cells will be killed by the persistence of the active drug on the peritoneal lining. Supporting evidence for this hypothesis is provided by the observation in one experimental system that tumor cells implanted into the peritoneal cavity up to 30 days following intraperitoneal mitoxantrone instillation are unable to grow, while the same tumor will easily take hold if administered by the intraperitoneal route without prior mitoxantrone administration (Murdock et al., 1985).

In the Phase 1 trials objective antitumor responses, including decreases of abnormal CA-125 levels into the normal range in refractory ovarian carcinoma, have been observed.

In the several reported Phase 1 studies, abdominal pain was felt to be mild or moderate in severity with a single mitoxantrone dose of 25 to 30 mg/m^2 (delivered in 2 l of normal saline). Beyond this dose level severe pain was noted. However, in a recently completed Phase 2 trial of intraperitoneal mitoxantrone in refractory ovarian cancer conducted at the Memorial Sloan-Kettering Cancer Center, severe abdominal pain was observed in the majority of patients treated with a single dose of 30 mg/m^2, and at the 20-mg/m^2 dose level most individuals required narcotic analgesia at some point during their treatment course (Markman, George, et al., 1990). Of greater concern were the findings at response laparotomy where extensive adhesion formation was noted in almost all patients (whether treated at 20 or 30 mg/m^2). Four of the 31 patients entered into this trial experienced episodes of bowel obstruction during therapy while an additional 2 patients required surgical intervention for obstruction and intra-abdominal abscess formation several months after the completion of therapy. This experience led the Sloan-Kettering investigators to conclude that the regimen employed produced unacceptable local toxicity, despite impressive clinical activity (see Section 4.7 in Chapter 4).

Several options have been proposed to reduce the severity of the local toxicity produced by mitoxantrone. Considering that all investigators examining the intraperitoneal administration of the agent have found minimal systemic toxicity, it might be possible to deliver the drug more frequently but at a lower concentration. This should reduce the irritant effects of the agent while at the same time maintaining or even increasing the dose intensity of mitoxantrone drug delivery. Alternatively, intraperitoneal mitoxantrone might be administered along with nonsteroidal anti-inflammatory agents. Under experimental conditions such drugs have been demonstrated to reduce the local toxicity associated with intraperitoneal chemotherapy administration (Markman, Vasilev, et al., 1986).

4.5.8 Melphalan and Thiotepa

Despite the earlier disappointing results with the intraperitoneal administration of alkylating agents, it was natural that there would be interest in reexploring the use of this category of drugs for intracavitary delivery because of their known activity in ovarian cancer (Thigpen et al., 1987). Several groups have examined the intraperitoneal administration of melphalan as a single agent (Holcenberg et al., 1983; Howell, Pfeifle, and Olshen, 1984). A significant pharmacokinetic advantage was observed (approximately 100-fold) for peritoneal cavity exposure with minimal local side effects. Dose-limiting toxicity was bone marrow suppression. Only marginal clinical activity was noted in patients with refractory ovarian cancer treated with intraperitoneal melphalan; however, this finding is not surprising in view of the known limited activity of aklylating agents in patients who have failed prior cisplatin-based treatment (Pater et al., 1987). It is certainly possible that greater efficacy might be observed in less heavily pretreated patients.

In view of the fact that the dose-limiting toxicity of intraperitoneal melphalan has been found to be bone marrow suppression, one could argue that the intraperitoneal route of drug delivery for this alkylating agent (as well as for other drugs such as cisplatin) would be preferred over intravenous administration in ovarian cancer, because systemic exposure (through capillary flow) is not compromised and local tumor–drug interactions are enhanced (uptake by free-surface diffusion). However, only through the conduct of randomized controlled clinical trials can the validity of this hypothesis be appropriately tested.

In two recently reported trials of intraperitoneal thiotepa, bone marrow suppression was found to be the dose-limiting toxicity (Kirmani et al., 1989; Wadler et al., 1989). Unfortunately, only a small pharmacokinetic advantage (fourfold) was demonstrated following the intraperitoneal delivery of this agent compared with systemic drug levels.

4.5.9 Mitomycin C

Mitomycin C is one of the more interesting standard chemotherapeutic agents to consider for intraperitoneal administration. The drug is commonly used as a second-line agent in a number of malignancies, including ovarian cancer (Thigpen et al., 1987). The Japanese have reported an extensive experience using intraperitoneal mitomycin as an adjuvant therapy following curative surgery for gastric cancer, but there is essentially no experience with this therapeutic approach in the United States (Douglass, 1985).

In several Phase 1 trials of intraperitoneal mitomycin C an impressive pharmacokinetic advantage for this route of drug delivery has been demonstrated (Table 4.1) (Adams, Patt, and Rosenblum, 1984; Gyves, 1985). Dose-limiting toxicity is abdominal pain and adhesion formation, particularly with dose levels exceeding 10 mg/m^2. Impressive activity for intraperitoneal mitomycin C has been noted in refractory ovarian cancer (Monk et al., 1988), and the drug has even been employed when delivered by this route as initial treatment of ovarian carcinoma (Fujiwara et al., 1989). Unfortunately, in view of the local toxicity observed following intraperitoneal delivery of the drug, it is not certain how the agent can or should be used in clinical practice. In addition, the development of significant adhesions will limit the number of courses of the agent that can be administered into the peritoneal cavity.

Because intraperitoneal mitomycin C causes little bone marrow suppression, one reported approach to employing the agent has been to alternate the drug given in relatively low doses (5 to 10 mg) with intraperitoneal cisplatin in the treatment of peritoneal mesothelioma (Markman et al., 1989).

4.5.10 Bleomycin

As previously noted, intracavitary bleomycin has been used for many years as an approach to prevent malignant fluid reaccumulation, particularly malignant pleural effusion (Ostrowski, 1986; Ostrowski and Halsall, 1982). Somewhat less successful have been the efforts to use single-agent intraperitoneal bleomycin to control malignant ascites (Ostrowski and Halsall, 1982). Because there is evidence of synergy between cisplatin and bleomycin, defined both clinically (Einhorn and Donohue, 1977) and experimentally (Mascharak et al., 1983), as well as activity for the drug in ovarian cancer (Blackledge et al., 1984), it was reasonable to consider further exploration of a role for bleomycin as a cytotoxic agent when administered by the intraperitoneal route. Three groups have defined a significant pharmacokinetic advantage for intraperitoneal bleomycin delivery (Table 4.1) (Alberts, Chen, et al., 1979; Bitran, 1985; Howell, Schiefer, et al., 1987). Local toxicity was observed, and systemic side effects including fever and chills were common. Unfortunately, there was little evidence of a therapeutic benefit in the single-agent Phase 1 trials, other than a decrease in malignant fluid reaccumulation.

4.5.11 Cytarabine

Cytarabine is a cell-cycle-specific agent that has demonstrated very limited evidence of activity in solid tumors (Wasserman et al., 1975). However, it can be argued that the drug has not been optimally used in this clinical setting because of the concern for producing profound bone marrow suppression with prolonged infusions. Because cytarabine is rapidly and extensively metabolized by the liver during its first passage through that organ, it is not surprising that there exists nearly a 3-log advantage for peritoneal cavity exposure to the drug compared with the systemic circulation following direct intraperitoneal instillation (Table 4.1) (King, Pfeifle, and Howell, 1984; Markman, 1985; Markman and Howell, 1985a).

In a small clinical study the local toxicity of single-agent intraperitoneal cytarabine was found to be limited (King, Pfeifle, and Howell, 1984). Unfortunately, in this trial, patients were treated by dialysis exchange four times each day for 5 days and a high incidence of bacterial peritonitis was encountered. Dose-limiting toxicity was bone marrow suppression. Of interest, two patients with microscopic residual disease at the initiation of therapy became clinically disease free (peritoneal cavity cytologies converted from positive to negative) and remained in this clinical state for more than 3 years.

4.5.12 Streptozotocin

Streptozotocin, a chemotherapeutic agent with demonstrated activity in several malignancies, including colon carcinoma (Kemeny, 1987), has been administered by the intraperitoneal route to a single patient with a 100-fold pharmacokinetic advantage for cavity exposure being reported (Panasci et al., 1982). Although this finding requires confirmation, the possibility exists that streptozotocin might be considered for inclusion in a combination intraperitoneal program along with 5-FU or FUDR as an adjuvant chemotherapy regimen for colon carcinoma.

4.5.13 Etoposide and Teniposide

Etoposide (VP-16), one of the newest additions to the medical oncologist's armamentarium, has been examined for intraperitoneal administration by several groups (Allen et al., 1982; Daugherty et al., 1987; Fanning, Daugherty, and Weese, 1989; Littlewood, Lydon, and Booth, 1988; Zimm et al., 1987). In contrast to most of the chemotherapeutic agents previously considered for intraperitoneal delivery, etoposide is highly protein bound. Thus, the pharmacokinetic properties of the agent when administered by the intraperitoneal route exhibit somewhat unique properties. The advantage of cavity exposure to total (free plus protein bound) etoposide; is only fourfold. However, when considering only *free* (not protein bound) etoposide, the AUC for the peritoneal cavity is 64-fold higher than that of the systemic compartment (Zimm et al., 1987).

There are conflicting data as to the activity of single-agent systemically delivered etoposide in refractory ovarian cancer, but most investigators consider it to be a relatively inactive agent (Edmondson et al., 1978; Slayton et al., 1979). Therefore, clinical responses observed in the small reported trial of single-agent intraperitoneal etoposide in refractory ovarian carcinoma are of interest (Daugherty et al., 1987). Dose-limiting toxicity of intraperitoneal etoposide appears to be bone marrow suppression, with limited local toxicity being observed. This finding is of considerable importance because in one preclinical model system the intraperitoneal administration of etoposide was associated with severe local fibrous tissue formation (Stahelin, 1976).

The intraperitoneal administration of teniposide (VP-26) has been examined in a pilot study involving 18 patients with malignant ascites. Although only modest clinical activity was observed (control of ascites formation in several patients), the agent was reasonably well tolerated locally, and a 10-fold increased exposure of the peritoneal cavity to the agent compared with the plasma was demonstrated (Canal et al., 1989).

4.5.14 Combination intraperitoneal chemotherapy

Combination chemotherapy has been shown to improve the response rate and survival of a number of malignancies, including ovarian carcinoma (Einhorn and Donohue, 1977; Young et al., 1978). Therefore, it is not surprising that clinical investigators at a number of centers have begun to explore the potential of combination intraperitoneal therapy.

There are several attractive aspects of this therapeutic approach. First, as suggested in modeling studies, the emergence of drug resistance may be inhibited (Goldie and Coldman, 1979; Goldie, Coldman, and Gudauskas, 1982). Second, far higher concentrations of drugs can be safely attained within the peritoneal cavity than can be achieved following systemic drug delivery. Concentration-dependent cytotoxic synergy between chemotherapeutic agents has been demonstrated in vitro in several experimental systems (Markman, 1985, 1986). Thus, the intraperitoneal route of drug delivery allows for the testing of the clinical relevance of these provocative experimental observations in a manner not possible with systemic drug administration.

One note of caution must be voiced when considering combination intraperitoneal therapy. Although individual components of the proposed regimen may have been shown to produce acceptable local toxicity when delivered by the intraperitoneal route, it is possible that the combination may produce severe local effects. This consideration is somewhat unique to intracavitary drug delivery because the drugs will be together in solution and in contact with the cavity lining for considerable periods of time, often exceeding several hours. Subtle changes in the acid–base composition of the fluid or chemical structure of one of the agents (from drug–drug interactions) may, in theory, result in serious consequences (local pain or inflammation leading to extensive adhesion formation). Therefore, each new combination considered for intraperitoneal delivery must be carefully evaluated to define its safety. Now that intraperitoneal chemotherapy is beginning to be used commonly in clinical practice, it is important to reemphasize that the potential toxicity of this approach cannot be underestimated (Alberts et al., 1980; Markman et al., 1984; Markman, George, et al., 1990).

A number of Phase 1 combination cisplatin-based intraperitoneal programs have been examined, including cisplatin and cytarabine (Markman, Howell, et al., 1985); cisplatin, cytarabine, and doxorubicin (Markman et al., 1984); cisplatin, cytarabine, and bleomycin (Markman, Cleary, Lucas, et al., 1986; Piver et al., 1988); cisplatin and etoposide (Zimm et al., 1987); cisplatin and melphalan (Piccart et al., 1988); and cisplatin and 5-FU (Doroshow et al., 1986; Reichman et al., 1989b). These programs have been principally directed toward the development of clinically active intraperitoneal regimens in refractory ovarian cancer. Responses, including surgically defined complete responses, have been observed. However, it remains uncertain if the activity demonstrated in any of these trials is superior to that which would have been found with single-agent intraperitoneal cisplatin.

Toxicity has varied considerably with the different cisplatin-based intraperitoneal programs. Severe abdominal pain and adhesion formation were noted when doxorubicin was included in the intraperitoneal program. Bleomycin was also associated with pain, but of somewhat reduced severity compared with doxorubicin. The cisplatin and cytarabine regimen appeared to cause more pain than single-agent cisplatin, and adhesion formation was at times extensive. In addition, fever (presumably secondary to cytarabine) was noted in many patients. This was a disturbing side effect because distinguishing mild drug-induced peritoneal irritation with fever from an infectious peritonitis in a patient with an indwelling catheter can be difficult. Cisplatin and 5-FU combination therapy appeared to be reasonably well tolerated, except for moderate 5-FU-induced adhesion formation. Finally, the cisplatin and etoposide and cisplatin and melphalan regimens were reported to be well tolerated in most patients, with dose-limiting toxicity being bone marrow suppression.

On the basis of both preclinical and clinical data suggesting important synergistic activity between 5-FU or FUDR and leucovorin (Grem et al., 1987), several groups have begun to explore these drug combinations for intraperitoneal administration (Arbuck et al., 1986; Budd et al., 1986; Smith et al., 1989). Limited Phase 1 data would suggest the drugs are compatible in solution in the peritoneal cavity and the addition of leucovorin does not appear to increase the local toxicity produced by either 5-FU or FUDR. Of considerable interest, it appears that the levels of leucovorin demonstrated in experimental systems to be required to produce synergistic cytotoxicity with the pyrimidines can easily be achieved following intraperitoneal administration (Arbuck et al., 1986; Smith et al., 1989).

Clinical activity for these drug combinations, including surgically defined responses, has been observed in patients with small-volume intra-abdominal metastatic disease from gastrointestinal primary tumors. This approach has its greatest theoretical potential as adjuvant treatment of patients with gastrointestinal primary tumors at high risk of developing recurrent disease following curative resections.

4.5.15 Intraperitoneal therapy with biologic agents

There has been considerable recent interest in the intraperitoneal administration of biologic agents, based on data generated from trials of systemic delivery of the drugs and in vitro experimental evidence suggesting concentration-dependent cytotoxicity for a number of biologic agents against various malignancies (Eggermont, 1989; Markman, 1987a; Rosenberg, 1986). In addition, preclinical evaluation suggesting concentration-dependent synergy between biologic agents lends further support to the concept of regional drug delivery (Markman, 1987a). A final rationale for the intraperitoneal administration of biologic agents is the theoretical possibility that local immuno-regulatory mechanisms present within the cavity may be stimulated by the high concentrations of drug(s) to produce an antineoplastic effect.

A number of biologic agents have been reported to be administered by the intraperitoneal route as treatment of malignant disease (Eggermont, 1989; Markman, 1987a). The earliest work employed nonspecific immuno-stimulants, including Bacillus Clamette-Guerin, *Corynebacterium parvum,* and a streptococcal preparation (OK-432) (Bast et al., 1983; Berek, Knapp, et al., 1985; Katano and Torisu, 1983; Mantovani et al., 1981; Torisu et al., 1983). Clinical activity was observed when these agents were administered by the intraperitoneal route. However, local toxicity was often severe.

With the biologic agents made by recombinant DNA techniques available, it has been possible to test products that may produce a greater anti-neoplastic effect and less local inflammation. Perhaps the most interesting study to date has been the work of investigators at the University of California, Los Angeles, who administered recombinant alpha-interferon to a small group of patients with refractory ovarian carcinoma (Berek, Hacker, et al., 1985). Surgically defined complete responses were observed in four of seven patients with either microscopic disease only or no tumor nodule greater than 0.5 cm. Two small positive confirmatory studies have recently been reported from the Netherlands and South Africa (Bezwoda, Seymour, and Dansey, 1989; Willemse et al., 1989). Antineoplastic activity in this clinical setting for beta- (Rambaldi et al., 1985) and gamma-interferon (Pujade-Lauraine et al., 1990) has also been noted, but an earlier trial of intraperitoneal gamma-interferon failed to demonstrate objective responses (D'Acquisto et al., 1988). Although local toxicity with the intraperitoneal administration of the various interferons is observed (abdominal pain), it appears to be less than that seen with the nonspecific immunostimulants.

Antineoplastic activity has also been described when intraperitoneal interleukin-2 is administered with or without lymphokine-activated killer cells (Beller et al., 1989; Kamada et al., 1989; Lembersky et al., 1989; Lotze, Custer, and Rosenberg, 1986). However, when lymphokine-activated killer cells are employed local toxicity has been substantial (severe abdominal pain and adhesion formation).

The pharmacokinetic findings associated with the intraperitoneal administration of several biologic agents are of considerable interest. Preclinical modeling studies had previously suggested that large drugs, such as biologic agents, would be more slowly cleared from the peritoneal cavity than the much smaller chemotherapeutic agents because of their slow entry into the local capillary network (Dedrick, 1985). Actual clinical data have confirmed the predictions made by these modeling studies with substantial concentrations of alpha-interferon (Berek, Hacker, et al., 1985), interleukin-2 (Chapman et al., 1988), and tumor necrosis factor (Markman et al., 1989), persisting within the cavity more than 24 hours following intraperitoneal drug instillation. These data should be contrasted with the peritoneal cavity half-lives of several hours or less for most chemotherapeutic agents when delivered by the intraperitoneal route.

Finally, a number of investigators have directed their research efforts to defining a role for the intraperitoneal delivery of monoclonal antibodies, as both immunodiagnostic and immunotherapeutic tools (Markman, 1987a). Experimentally, it has been shown that certain radiolabeled monoclonal antibodies administered by the intraperitoneal route can more reliably detect intra-abdominal tumors than can the same antibody administered intravenously (Colcher et al., 1987; Haisma et al., 1988; Rowlinson et al., 1987; Yang and Reisfeld, 1988). Trials examining the potential clinical utility of this technique are under way at a number of centers.

Several groups have recently reported on their experience using radiolabeled monoclonal antibodies delivered by the intraperitoneal route as therapy for tumors confined to the peritoneal cavity (Epenetos, 1984, 1985; Epenetos et al., 1987; Finkler et al., 1989; Stewart et al., 1989; Ward et al., 1988). Objective antitumor responses have been observed and it has been suggested that these responses were directly related to the use of the antibody plus radioisotope.

However, caution must be exercised in interpreting the results of these and other trials employing intraperitoneal radiolabeled antibodies as therapy for intra-abdominal tumors, because it has long been established that the intraperitoneal administration of radioisotopes alone (without antibody) can be an effective form of cytotoxic antineoplastic therapy (Ariel, Oropeza, and Pack, 1966; Julian, Inalsingh, and Burnett, 1978; Piver et al., 1982). Despite this reservation, the intraperitoneal administration of tumor-related monoclonal antibodies attached to isotopes or biologic toxins, such as ricin or *Pseudomonas* endotoxin (Fer et al., 1989), has the potential to be an important therapeutic modality in patients with small-volume residual ovarian cancer or as an adjuvant treatment of gastrointestinal malignancies.

4.6 Innovative trials employing the intraperitoneal route

Because of the unique anatomic, physiologic, and pharmacologic properties of the peritoneal cavity, a number of investigators have developed interesting and highly innovative approaches to the management of malignant disease involving this region of the body. A number of preclinical and Phase 1 trials have been reported, the goals of which are briefly summarized below:

1. Modulation of the activity of intraperitoneally administered methotrexate by the addition of intraperitoneal dipyridamole, an inhibitor of nucleoside transport that has been demonstrated in an experimental system to increase the cytotoxicity of methotrexate in a concentration-dependent manner (Chan et al., 1988; Goel et al., 1989).

2. Intraperitoneal hyperthermic chemotherapy employing thiotepa and methotrexate (Spratt, Adcock, Muskovin, et al., 1980), mitomycin (Fujimoto et al., 1989; Harari et al., 1989; Koga et al., 1988), or cisplatin (Harari et al., 1989), based on preclinical data suggesting increased cytotoxicity of certain antineoplastic agents when employed in a hyperthermic environment (Dietzel, 1983; Hahn, 1979; Shiu and Fortner, 1980; Spratt, Adcock, Sherrill, et al., 1980; Stratford et al., 1980). This approach has also been applied experimentally in canines using intraperitoneal cisplatin (Zakris et al., 1987). It should be noted that severe renal

insufficiency developed in a single patient treated with intraperitoneal cisplatin (50 mg/m^2) and hyperthermia (Harari et al., 1989).

3. Whole-abdominal radiotherapy plus intraperitoneal radiosensitizing agents (misonidazole and demethylmisonidazole), designed to increase the efficacy and decrease the toxicity of the sensitizing agents (Gianni et al., 1983).

4. Prolonged continuous intraperitoneal administration of the antimetabolite thioguanine, designed to increase local exposure while reducing systemic toxicity (Zimm et al., 1988).

5. Preclinical investigation of the intraperitoneal administration of hexamethylmelamine, an active agent in ovarian carcinoma with limited solubility in aqueous solution (Thigpen et al., 1987), in a lipid-soluble vehicle (Intralipid) (Wickes and Howell, 1985).

6. Preclinical evaluation of a hematoporphyrin derivative and intraperitoneal laser light, designed to treat local tumor within the reach of the delivered light (Tochner et al., 1985).

7. Intraperitoneal chemotherapy with doxorubicin (Delgado et al., 1989) and cytarabine (Kim and Howell, 1987), entrapped within liposomes, designed to both increase the duration of cavity exposure and decrease local toxicity.

8. Intraperitoneal administration of medroxyprogesterone acetate (Camaggi et al., 1985), based on limited clinical data suggesting a dose response of advanced refractory ovarian carcinoma to progestational agents (Geisler, 1983).

9. Intraoperative or immediately postoperative intraperitoneal chemotherapy designed to optimize drug distribution and ensure that all areas of potential tumor involvement are bathed at least once prior to the establishment of intra-abdominal adhesions (Fujimoto et al., 1988; Hagiwara et al., 1988; Markman, Weiss, et al., 1985; Sugarbaker et al., 1988; Werner et al., 1989).

4.7 Efficacy trials of intraperitoneal chemotherapy in refractory ovarian cancer

Single-agent intraperitoneal cisplatin as treatment of refractory ovarian cancer has been examined in several Phase 2 clinical trials (Cohen, 1985; Hacker et al., 1987; Ten Bokkel Huinink et al., 1985). Overall, approximately 25 to 30 percent of the patients with small-volume residual refractory ovarian cancer participating in these trials experienced a surgically defined complete response. Unfortunately, the definition of refractory disease has varied in the small reported series. For example, patients whose disease had previously responded to intravenous cisplatin and then recurred, sometimes with a long treatment-free interval, have been considered together with patients who recently received intravenous cisplatin and either failed to respond or demonstrated only a partial response to the systemic treatment program. In addition, in the earliest reported Phase 2 intraperitoneal cisplatin trials, patients were included who had previously received alkylating agents (with or without doxorubicin) and not systemically administered cisplatin.

Responses to intravenous cisplatin are observed in approximately 20 to 50 percent of patients with ovarian cancer who have previously been treated with a non-cisplatin-containing regimen (Alberts, Hilger, et al., 1979; Neijt et al., 1984; Surwit et al., 1983; Vogl et al., 1982). In addition, patients with a number of malignancies, including ovarian cancer, who have demonstrated a response to a chemotherapy program but who relapse following a prolonged treatment-free period (usually more than 1 year) are known to have a high likelihood of responding again to the same or similar treatment regimen (Batist et al., 1983; Fisher et al., 1979; Markman, Rothman, et al., 1990; McVie et al., 1989; Seltzer, Vogl, and Kaplan, 1985). Thus, it is probably inappropriate to refer to such patients as having "refractory disease." The term "refractory ovarian cancer" should be reserved for patients who either have not responded to a cisplatin/carboplatin-based regimen or have demonstrated only a minor or partial response to such treatment. The delivery of additional systemic chemotherapy to such individuals shortly after the documentation of their failure to achieve a complete response has a less than 10 percent chance of producing that surgically defined result (Bertelsen et al., 1989; Hakes et al., 1987; Stiff, Lanzotti, and Roddick, 1983).

An additional difficulty with the early Phase 2 reports of single-agent cisplatin in refractory ovarian cancer is the fact that some patients were evaluated for response only by laparoscopy. Complete responses defined by this technique might have been found to be only partial, minor, or no response had a formal laparotomy been performed. Finally, the bulk of disease present at the initiation of treatment was not optimally defined in the literature reports. Thus, it is difficult to compare the surgically defined response rates of the single-agent cisplatin intraperitoneal trials to the more recent Phase 2 reports of intraperitoneal chemotherapy (i.e., combination cisplatin

Exhibit 4.1

Summary of Results of Phase 2 Trials of Intraperitoneal Cisplatin-based Therapy in Refractory Ovarian Cancer

Overall surgically defined response rate: 20–30 percent

Surgically defined response rate with largest tumor mass measuring 0.5 cm or less in diameter: 40–50 percent

Surgically defined response rate with tumor nodules greater than 0.5 cm: less than 10–20 percent

based or mitoxantrone chemotherapy), which have provided far greater details of tumor volumes at treatment initiation.

Several Phase 2 cisplatin-based intraperitoneal regimens have been reported with surgically defined complete remission being observed principally in patients whose largest tumor mass measured less than 0.5 to 1 cm in diameter (Exhibit 4.1). Overall, keeping in mind the reservations discussed above, the response rates in the Phase 2 cisplatin-based combination chemotherapy programs have been similar to those observed with single-agent cisplatin (approximately 30 percent). However, it should be noted that in individuals with very small tumor nodules (0.5 cm or less) or microscopic disease only, the surgically defined response rate (complete and partial) approaches 50 percent (Piver et al., 1988; Reichman et al., 1989a, 1990).

One of the key unanswered questions concerning cisplatin-based intraperitoneal therapy for refractory ovarian cancer is whether the percentage of complete responses observed is superior to what would have been seen if patients demonstrating a partial response to systemically delivered cisplatin had been continued on the same or a similar intravenous regimen. In the absence of a randomized trial addressing this important point; it is possible to provide a preliminary assessment of the relative benefits (if any) of intraperitoneal cisplatin by comparing the results of such treatment with those limited clinical trials in which patients achieving a partial response following five or six cycles of systemic treatment were continued on an additional five or six courses of systemic cisplatin and subsequently underwent a planned laparotomy to determine if they were in a complete remission.

Three trials have been identified in the oncology literature that fulfill these criteria (Bertelsen et al., 1989; Hakes et al., 1987; Stiff, Lanzotti, and Roddick, 1983). Of the 35 patients treated in this manner, 3 (9 percent) achieved a complete remission with continued systemic cisplatin-based treatment. Five second-line single-agent cisplatin and combination cisplatin-based intraperitoneal programs of small-volume refractory ovarian carcinoma have been reported that provide sufficient information to allow a reasonable comparison with the intravenous studies (Cohen, 1985; Ten Bokkel Huinink et al., 1985; Hacker et al., 1987; Piver et al., 1988; Reichman et al., 1989a). Thirty-three of the 122 patients (27 percent) treated on these five trials achieved a surgically documented complete response. This difference is statistically significant at the $p < 0.025$ level (chi-square test, 1 degree of freedom).

One must be cautious in the interpretation of these data because in this evaluation of nonrandomized trials it is uncertain if patient characteristics such as tumor grade, prechemotherapy stage, and bulk of disease present at the initiation of intraperitoneal treatment were comparable between the two groups. However, in the absence of a randomized trial comparing the treatment approaches, this analysis suggests the superiority of intraperitoneal cisplatin-based treatment in the setting of small-volume residual/refractory ovarian cancer.

In a Phase 2 trial of single-agent intraperitoneal carboplatin in refractory ovarian cancer conducted by the Northern California Oncology Group, a response rate (complete and partial) of 23 percent for the patients with measurable disease was documented (Scudder et al., 1989). This activity for single-agent intraperitoneal carboplatin in refractory ovarian cancer has been confirmed in an ongoing trial being conducted at the New York University Medical Center (Colombo et al., 1987).

Investigators at the National Cancer Institute conducted a Phase 2 trial of intraperitoneal 5-FU in 14 patients with refractory ovarian cancer, 12 of whom had previously received the drug delivered by the intravenous route (Ozols, Speyer, et al., 1984). Only 1 patient (7 percent) responded, but this response was a surgically defined complete remission in one of the 2 patients who had not had prior exposure to 5-FU. Although this agent is now rarely used in front-line chemotherapy programs for ovarian cancer, it is possible the drug may demonstrate greater activity in patients who have failed their initial chemotherapy regimen.

In a Phase 2 trial of intraperitoneal mitoxantrone conducted at the Memorial Sloan-Kettering Cancer Center, 6 of 18 patients (33 percent) whose large tumor diameter measured less than 1 cm at protocol entry demonstrated a surgically-defined response (4 complete responses) (Markman, George, et al., 1990). Only 1 of 11 patients (9 percent) with a single tumor mass greater than 1 cm responded to the treatment program. Of considerable interest, several of the responding patients had previously demonstrated unequivocal progression or failure to respond to intraperitoneal cisplatin. However, as previously discussed, this impressive response rate must be viewed in the context of the potential for serious local toxicity associated with the intraperitoneal administration of mitoxantrone.

4.8 Efficacy studies of intraperitoneal therapy in peritoneal mesothelioma

Three groups have reported their experience employing intraperitoneal therapy as part of a management program for peritoneal mesothelioma. The approach of the Dana-Farber Cancer Center has been to combine aggressive surgical debulking with intraperitoneal cisplatin and doxorubicin and whole-abdominal radiotherapy (Antman et al., 1985). Compared with an institutional historical control population, the small number of patients treated with this intensive therapeutic approach have demonstrated an impressive improvement in survival (with 6 of 10 patients free of disease 19 + to 78 + months following diagnosis) (Lederman et al., 1987). The specific contribution of the intraperitoneal therapy to the clinical utility of this multimodality program is uncertain, but the extensive surgical debulking does allow small-volume residual tumor to come into direct contact with the high concentrations of the cytotoxic drugs.

Investigators at the UCSD Cancer Center (Pfeifle, Howell, and Markman, 1985; Markman, Cleary, Pfeifle, et al., 1986) and the Memorial Sloan-Kettering Cancer Center (Markman and Kelsen, 1989) have focused their efforts on intraperitoneal cisplatin-based treatment. Control of malignant ascites and regression of tumor nodules (surgically documented) have been reported. In addition, several patients treated by this therapeutic approach have remained clinically disease free for more than 3 years from the initiation of treatment.

4.9 Efficacy studies of intraperitoneal therapy in gastrointestinal cancers

In 1985, investigators at the National Cancer Institute reported the results of a randomized trial of adjuvant intraperitoneal 5-FU versus intravenous 5-FU in patients with colon carcinoma who had a high risk of developing recurrent disease (Sugarbaker et al., 1985, 1986). Unfortunately, there was no untreated control population included in this trial. Although there was no difference in disease-free or overall survival in the two treatment groups, there was a statistically significant decrease in peritoneal cavity recurrences (determined at second-look laparotomy) in patients receiving the intraperitoneal 5-FU.

This would suggest that the high concentrations of 5-FU bathing the peritoneal cavity were capable of killing microscopic disease present in the cavity but the far lower concentrations achieved elsewhere were unable to inhibit tumor growth. An additional conclusion that may reasonably be drawn from this trial is that it is unlikely the enhanced local cytotoxic effect associated with intraperitoneal therapy can be translated into improved survival in gastrointestinal malignancies until more active chemotherapeutic agents for the diseases become available (Kemeny, 1987).

4.10 Summary and recommendations

Both preclinical and clinical evaluations have helped to define the situations in which intraperitoneal therapy is a reasonable therapeutic option for patients with malignant disease. A brief outline of the patient populations with ovarian and nonovarian cancers who might be considered for clinical trials

---

Exhibit 4.2

Ovarian Cancer: Appropriate Clinical Situations for Trials of Intraperitoneal Therapy

1. Patients with small-volume residual disease (microscopic, nodules 0.5 cm or less in diameter) following systemic therapy with or without secondary surgical debulking prior to intraperitoneal therapy;

2. Patients with high-grade tumors who experience a surgically defined complete response, but in whom the ultimate relapse rate approaches 50 percent (Copeland and Gershenson, 1986);

3. Initial therapy, with all drugs delivered by the intraperitoneal route (i.e., cisplatin and etoposide or carboplatin and etoposide);

4. Initial therapy, with certain drugs delivered intravenously (i.e., cyclophosphamide) and others by the intraperitoneal route (i.e., cisplatin and carboplatin);

5. Initial therapy as part of a program including a limited number of courses of intravenous drug delivery (with or without additional surgical debulking) followed by intraperitoneal therapy.

Exhibit 4.3

Nonovarian Malignancies: Appropriate Clinical Situations for Trials of Intraperitoneal Therapy

1. Patients with peritoneal mesothelioma (with or without an attempt at prior surgical debulking);

2. Patients with gastrointestinal cancer and documented positive peritoneal cytologies or random biopsies, or with very small tumor nodules (0.5 cm or less);

3. Adjuvant therapy of patients with gastrointestinal cancer with a higher risk of recurrence in the peritoneal cavity (i.e., gastric and colon cancer) following curative surgery.

---

of intraperitoneal therapy, based on our current knowledge of the technique, is presented in Exhibits 4.2 and 4.3.

Several groups have recently begun to explore the use of intraperitoneal cisplatin-based treatment as an integral part of initial treatment of advanced ovarian cancer (Hakes et al., 1989; Howell et al., 1990; Speyer et al., 1987; Zambetti et al., 1989). Randomized trials will be required to determine if the pharmacokinetic advantage associated with intraperitoneal therapy can be translated into a survival benefit for patients treated with this therapeutic approach.

Similarly, in the absence of data from randomized trials, it is difficult to know if the clinically defined or surgically defined responses to intraperitoneal therapy in refractory ovarian cancer have been or will be translated into a survival benefit for the patients treated by this approach. Several groups have noted prolonged survival for patients with small-volume residual ovarian cancer treated with cisplatin-based intraperitoneal therapy (Howell, Zimm, et al., 1987; Menczer et al., 1989). However, it is uncertain whether these observations reflect a true benefit for this approach or merely the well-recognized natural history of long-term survival for a subset of patients with known small-volume residual disease following initial chemotherapy (Copeland et al., 1985; Hoskins et al., 1989; Neijt et al., 1986; Podratz et al., 1988; Wharton, Edwards, and Rutledge, 1984).

For the present, and on the basis of Phase 1 and 2 trials of intraperitoneal therapy, it appears appropriate to draw the following conclusions:

1. Intraperitoneal treatment with single-agent cisplatin or carboplatin or a cisplatin- or carboplatin-based regimen is at least equivalent and may be

superior to alternative treatment options in patients with ovarian cancer who have responded to a systemically delivered cisplatin- or carboplatin-based regimen but continue to have very small volume disease remaining at the completion of the intravenous program.

2. Other drugs that have demonstrated activity in small-volume residual ovarian cancer, including mitoxantrone and alpha-interferon, are reasonable therapeutic options in patients who cannot be treated with a cisplatin- or carboplatin-based intraperitoneal program (i.e., previous nephrotoxicity, neurotoxicity, serious marrow suppression), or who have failed to demonstrate a response to a systemically delivered cisplatin or carboplatin regimen.

3. Unfortunately, in the absence of randomized trials comparing various intraperitoneal regimens, it is not possible to pick the best regimen for intraperitoneal treatment of small-volume refractory ovarian cancer (single-agent cisplatin, cisplatin-based combination therapy, mitoxantrone, alpha-interferon, etc.).

4. Patients with refractory ovarian cancer and tumor nodules greater than 1 cm rarely demonstrate objective evidence of a response to intraperitoneal cisplatin-based treatment. Such individuals should be considered for systemic treatment or other investigative programs.

5. Patients with peritoneal mesothelioma and a good performance status should be considered for an aggressive attempt at surgical debulking, followed by intraperitoneal therapy with a cisplatin-based program (with or without whole-abdominal radiotherapy).

6. Patients with documented small-volume implants from gastrointestinal malignancies and no obvious metastatic lesions in the liver can be considered for intraperitoneal therapy with a 5-FU- or FUDR-based program. Unfortunately, although this is a very reasonable therapeutic approach, there are currently no data available to demonstrate improved efficacy through the use of regional drug delivery in this clinical setting.

5 Intravesical Therapy for Superficial Bladder Cancer

5.1 Scope of the clinical issues and alternative treatment options

Approximately 47,000 new cases of bladder cancer are discovered in the United States each year (Silverberg and Lubera, 1989), 70 to 80 percent of which are found to be superficial at initial presentation (Soloway, 1984). Although these tumors are confined to the mucosa and submucosa of the bladder and are thus potentially curable by transurethral resection, 50 to 80 percent of patients will demonstrate recurrence within 3 to 5 years of local surgical resection (Soloway, 1980; Whitmore, 1979). Of greatest concern, 10 to 30 percent of patients will develop tumors of higher grade or stage, requiring more aggressive therapy (cystectomy, radiotherapy, or systemic chemotherapy).

The extremely high recurrence rate following surgical resection of low-grade tumors of the bladder is believed to be due to both the multifocal origin of cancers of the bladder and tumor implantation at the time of transurethral resection (Soloway and Murphy, 1979; Whitmore, 1979).

An important feature to note in a patient with localized bladder cancer is the histologic finding of carcinoma in situ. It is now recognized that this represents the early development of invasive cancer and suggests a diffuse abnormality in the bladder wall. Although radical cystectomy is curative, less aggressive treatment options of reasonable therapeutic potential would obviously be preferable (Utz et al., 1980).

5.2 Rationale for intravesical therapy for superficial bladder cancer

For several reasons early-stage bladder cancer is an attractive clinical situation to approach with regional (intravesical) antineoplastic drug administration (Exhibit 5.1). First, as noted above, the tumor is superficial at initial

Exhibit 5.1

Rationale for Intravesical Therapy for Superficial Bladder Cancer

1. Superficial tumor growth at presentation;
2. Ability to remove all macroscopic tumor in most patients;
3. Availability of active cytotoxic agents in bladder cancer;
4. Potential for frequent local instillations;
5. Ability to monitor closely the results of local therapy.

presentation in the majority of patients (Soloway, 1984). Second, in most individuals it is possible to surgically remove all macroscopic tumor, leaving only microscopic disease to be treated by the antineoplastic agents (Whitmore, 1979). Third, a number of cytotoxic agents have demonstrated activity in bladder cancer and might be considered for intravesical therapy (Knuchel et al., 1989; Yagoda, 1987). Finally, the bladder is easily accessible for frequent treatment instillations (Soloway, 1988a). This also makes it possible to assess the efficacy of intravesical treatment, as well as to discover at a relatively early time that local therapy has failed and alternative strategies are indicated.

5.3 Clinical trials of intravesical therapy

Drugs selected for intravesical therapy would ideally possess the following characteristics:

1. Significant antineoplastic activity against urothelial tumors;
2. Demonstrated limited absorption into the systemic circulation (to minimize systemic toxicity);
3. Production of little or no irritation of the bladder mucosa.

On the basis of these considerations, a number of chemotherapeutic and biologic agents have been examined for their safety and clinical activity following intravesical therapy, both as treatment of known residual superficial bladder cancer and as adjunctive therapy following complete surgical tumor removal (Exhibit 5.2) (Torti and Lum, 1984). In this latter situation treatment is administered to prevent tumor recurrence. Summarized below are

Exhibit 5.2

Antineoplastic Agents with Demonstrated Efficacy following Intravesical Administration in the Management of Superficial Bladder Cancer

Thiotepa	Bacillus Calmette-Guerin
Mitomycin C	Alpha-interferon
Doxorubicin	

Exhibit 5.3

Selected Regimens for Intravesical Therapy for Superficial Bladder Cancer

Thiotepa: 30 mg in 30 ml of saline weekly for 6–8 weeks, then monthly

Mitomycin C: 40 mg in 30–40 ml of saline weekly for 8 weeks

Doxorubicin: 50 mg in 60 ml of saline for 6 weeks, then monthly

Bacillus Calmette-Guerin: 1 ampule in 50–60 ml of saline weekly for 6 weeks

the results of clinical trials of intravesical therapy for superficial bladder cancer (also see Exhibit 5.3).

5.3.1 Thiotepa

Thiotepa has been used for intravesical therapy for bladder cancer for more than 25 years (Jones and Swinney, 1961). The agent has been used both as treatment of residual tumors and as prophylactic therapy to prevent tumor recurrence (Jones and Swinney, 1961; Koontz et al., 1981; Prout et al., 1983; Veenema et al., 1969). In one experimental system it has been demonstrated that the administration of thiotepa prior to tumor growth may retard the progression of low- to high-grade tumors (Soloway and Murphy, 1979).

Approximately 40 to 60 percent of patients with residual tumors following transureteral resection will respond to the intravesical administration of thiotepa, particularly those with low-grade tumors (Koontz et al., 1981;

Soloway, 1984). In several prophylactic trials, thiotepa decreased the relapse rate at 2-year follow-up from 70 percent (untreated control population) to 40 to 50 percent (Koontz et al., 1981; Prout et al., 1983; Netto and Lemos, 1983, Soloway, 1984).

A number of treatment regimens employing intravesical thiotepa have been investigated in clinical trials, but a dose of 30 mg administered in 30 ml of saline on a weekly schedule for 6 to 8 weeks, followed by monthly treatment as indicated, appears equally effective to higher dose regimens (Koontz et al., 1981).

Thiotepa is generally well tolerated locally with mild irritative voiding symptoms, with the dose-limiting side effect being bone marrow suppression (Hollister and Coleman, 1980; Soloway and Ford, 1983).This is due to the fact that the agent has a low molecular weight and enters the systemic compartment in significant concentrations following intravesical administration. In addition, several patients have been described who developed hematologic malignancies following prolonged intravesical thiotepa therapy (Hollister and Coleman, 1980). Finally, several cases of a rare benign tumor (nephrogenic adenoma) have been reported to develop following intravesical thiotepa (Wood, Streem, and Levin, 1988).

5.3.2 Mitomycin C

A number of investigators have examined the clinical activity of mitomycin C when delivered by the intravesical route in the management of superficial bladder cancer (Bracken et al., 1980; Huland et al., 1984; Issell et al., 1984; Kim and Lee, 1989; Mishina et al., 1975; Prout et al., 1982; Tolley et al., 1988). Overall, 60 to 70 percent of patients treated with the local administration of this agent have responded, with a complete response rate of 35 to 45 percent (Bracken et al., 1980; Mishina et al., 1975). Of considerable interest, patients who have failed intravesical thiotepa therapy can respond to the local administration of mitomycin C (Issell et al., 1984; Prout et al., 1982). The agent also has major activity in carcinoma in situ of the bladder, with one report noting that of 19 patients with this condition treated with intravesical mitomycin C, 15 achieved a complete response (Stricker et al., 1987).

Intravesical mitomycin C also appears to influence the rate of tumor recurrence and survival when administered prophylactically. In one study the recurrence rate following intravesical mitomycin C was 10 percent, compared with a 50 percent recurrence rate in the untreated control population (Huland et al., 1984). In addition, in this trial, the 2.5-year survival rate for the mitomycin C-treated patients was 100 percent compared with 84 percent for the untreated patients. Of note, one recently reported randomized study involving only 43 patients has failed to demonstrate an advantage for the prophylactic use of intravesical mitomycin C (Kim and Less, 1989).

As with thiotepa, several intravesical mitomycin C regimens have been investigated. A dose of 40 mg in 30 to 40 ml of saline administered weekly for 8 weeks appears to be a reasonably well tolerated treatment program (Issell et al., 1984; Soloway, 1984). There are also data available that suggest that multiple treatments with intravesical mitomycin C are superior to a single instillation (Tolley et al., 1988) and selected patients appear to benefit from maintenance treatment (Van Der Meijden and DeBruyne, 1988).

Little mitomycin C is absorbed into the systemic ciculation following local bladder administration (Wajsman et al., 1984), and marrow suppression is generally not observed (Mishina et al., 1975; Nissenkorn, Herrod, and Soloway, 1981). Local side effects, including urinary frequency and painful urination, develop in approximately 25 percent of treated patients (Nissenkorn, Herrod, and Soloway, 1981). However, severe contraction of the bladder following intravesical mitomycin C therapy has been described (Wajsman et al., 1983). In addition, skin rashes following local drug therapy, presumed to be a contact dermatitis, have been observed (Nissenkorn, Herrod, and Soloway, 1981).

5.3.3 Doxorubicin

Doxorubicin has been demonstrated to be a very active agent when administered by the intravesical route as therapy for superficial bladder cancer (Banks et al., 1977; Garnick et al., 1984; Lundbeck et al., 1988; Lundbeck, Mogensen, and Jeppesen, 1983). Of interest, there are limited data available to suggest that the agent may concentrate preferentially in small bladder tumors following local drug administration (Nakada et al., 1985). One trial reported a response rate of 86 percent in superficial bladder cancer, 52 percent of which were complete responses (Lundbeck, Mogensen, and Jeppesen, 1983).

There is essentially no absorption of doxorubicin into the systemic circulation, and systemic toxicity is not observed when the agent is administered directly into the bladder (Garnick et al., 1984; Jacobi and Kurth, 1980). The major toxicity is local (hematuria, dysuria, and urinary frequency).

One recommended dose of the agent for intravesical therapy is 50 mg in 60 ml of saline administered weekly for 6 weeks. Treatment may then be repeated monthly.

In an effort to decrease the recurrence rate following complete surgical removal of superficial bladder cancer, a recently reported study combined intravesical doxorubicin and mitomycin C (delivered at different times) as prophylactic therapy of resected patients (Ferraris, 1988). Unfortunately, the recurrence rate at 2 years (30 percent) was not different from what would have been expected with either agent administered alone in this clinical setting.

5.3.4 Cisplatin

There has been obvious interest in the use of cisplatin as a possible agent for intravesical therapy, because of its known activity when administered systemically as therapy of advanced bladder cancer (Yagoda, 1987) and its demonstrated safety and efficacy when administered into other body cavities (Markman, 1986). Unfortunately, the drug has limited activity when administered locally in the treatment of superficial bladder cancer and cannot be recommended for this purpose (Blumenreich et al., 1982).

5.3.5 Bacillus Calmette-Guerin

Bacillus Calmette-Guerin (BCG) was initially examined for intravesical administration as therapy for superficial bladder cancers in the mid-1970s (Morales, Eidinger, and Bruce, 1976). Both the early and subsequent reports have demonstrated that BCG has major clinical activity when delivered locally in this clinical setting (Guinan, Crispen, and Rubenstein, 1987).

The mechanism of BCG action is not totally understood; however, it is believed to produce its cytotoxic effect through immunologic mechanisms (Guinan, Crispen, and Rubenstein, 1987; Guinan, Shaw, and Ray, 1986; Prescott et al., 1989). Several reports have suggested that the antitumor activity of BCG is correlated with local interleukin-2 production (Fleischmann et al., 1989; Haaff, Catalona, and Batliff, 1986). (These provocative data have led investigators in Germany to treat a small group of patients with intravesical interleukin-2 in a small pilot study, with evidence of efficacy being demonstrated [Huland and Huland, 1989]).

In addition, several clinical trials have noted superior results in individuals who demonstrate a granulomatous inflammatory reaction in the bladder or who exhibit a positive skin test to purified protein derivative (PPD) (Kelley et al., 1985, 1986; Lamm, 1985; Lamm et al., 1982; Torrence et al., 1988; Van Der Meijden et al., 1989). In one report, 19 of 25 patients (77 percent) who converted from a negative skin test to a positive test remained free of tumor following intravesical BCG treatment, compared with only 11 of 32 individuals (34 percent) who failed to convert their skin test (Kelley et al., 1986). However, in a more recent report, the overall clinical significance of these findings has been questioned and it has been suggested that patient management decisions should not be based on whether or not a patient has a positive PPD skin test (Torrence et al., 1988).

Support for the intravesical use of BCG is also provided in the experimental setting using the mouse bladder tumor MBT-2 (Morales and Pang, 1986; Shapiro et al., 1984). In this system BCG has been shown to be more effective than intravesical thiotepa or mitomycin C in preventing tumor implantation following surgical removal of the malignancy (Shapiro et al., 1984).

Several clinical trials have confirmed that approximately 50 to 60 percent of patients with residual tumors following transureteral resection will achieve a complete response following BCG administration (Guinan, Crispen, and Rubenstein, 1987). In addition, the agent appears quite effective in preventing tumor recurrence following complete surgical removal of the malignancy (Guinan, Crispen, and Rubenstein, 1987; Herr et al., 1988; Lamm et al., 1981, 1982; Pinsky et al., 1985). Of great importance, treatment with BCG appears to reduce the ultimate requirement that a cystectomy be performed (Herr et al., 1988). It has also been noted that second responses to intravesical BCG occur in patients who initially experience a prolonged response to the local administration of the agent (Bretton et al., 1990). Finally, intravesical BCG can be effective therapy for superficial bladder cancer in patients who have failed treatment with intravesical thiotepa or mitomycin C (Schellhammer, Ladaga, and Fillion, 1986; Soloway and Perry, 1987).

Also of interest are reports of major activity for intravesical BCG in patients with carcinoma in situ of the bladder (Brosman, 1985; DeKernion et al., 1985; Herr et al., 1985, 1986; Kelley et al., 1985; Lamm, 1985; Mydlo et al., 1986; Schellhammer, Ladaga, and Fillion, 1986; Soloway, 1988b). Overall, 65 to 75 percent of patients with carcinoma in situ can be anticipated to achieve a complete response to this treatment strategy (Guinan, Crispen, and Rubenstein, 1987). However, appropriate caution in the use of intravesical therapy in the management of carcinoma in situ of the bladder has been advised because progression of the disease has been observed during intravesical chemotherapy and radical cystectomy can be highly curative in this clinical setting, if performed prior to tumor progression (Droller and Walsh, 1985).

Intravesical BCG is associated with a number of side effects, both local (hematuria, dysuria, urinary frequency, bladder contraction, ureteral obstruction, and granulomatous prostatitis) and systemic (fever, emesis, arthralgias, granulomatous hepatitis, and military tuberculosis) (Gupta, Lavengood, and Smith, 1988; Lamm et al., 1986; Linn, Klimberg, and Wajsman, 1989; Marans and Bekirov, 1987; Morales, 1984; Oates et al., 1988;

Steg et al., 1989). It has been suggested that the prophylactic administration of isoniazid can prevent both the serious local and systemic toxicities of treatment if administered for 3 days beginning on the day of intravesical treatment (Lamm et al., 1986).

Concern has also been raised for the possible development of second primaries, within the bladder, prostate, or other locations following intravesical BCG administration (Guinan et al., 1989; Hardeman, Perry, and Soloway, 1988; Khanna, Chou, et al., 1988). For the present, there appear to be only limited anecdotal data to support this concern, and the observed clinical utility of BCG would seem to outweigh any theoretical risk of the agent, including the induction of second primary cancers.

Five strains of BCG are available for clinical use, and several have been examined in the aforementioned clinical trials (Guinan, Crispen, and Rubenstein, 1987). At the present time it is not possible to make a definitive statement as to the preferred preparation for intravesical administration in the treatment of superficial bladder cancer. This is an important point because the viability of the BCG organism in the lot employed for therapy appears to strongly influence the likelihood of therapeutic success (Kelley et al., 1985). Fortunately, the recent approval by the U.S. Food and Drug Administration of a preparation of BCG for intravesical delivery greatly simplifies this issue.

In general, BCG has been administered weekly for approximately 6 weeks (Guinan, Crispen, and Rubenstein, 1987). One ampule is delivered in 50 to 60 ml of saline. A second treatment course may be successful if the first 6-week course fails to achieve a complete response (Kavoussi et al., 1988), but one report has suggested that with the failure of two courses alternative treatment options should be employed to prevent the risk of the development of invasive cancer (Catalona et al., 1987). The finding of either a positive or suspicious cytology following intravesical BCG treatment appears to be a good predictor of tumor recurrence (Badalament et al., 1987). Alternatively, flow cytometry of bladder washes obtained 6 months following BCG treatment has been successfully used to predict tumor recurrence (Bretton et al., 1989).

5.3.6 Alpha-interferon

The intravesical administration of recombinant alpha-interferon as therapy for superficial bladder cancer and carcinoma in situ has been examined by several groups (Ackermann et al., 1988; Torti et al., 1988; Williams, 1988). Approximately 30 percent of patients achieved a complete response, including patients previously treated with other intravesical treatments. In one study, 8 of 12 patients (67 percent) previously untreated with intravesical therapy achieved a complete or partial response to this treatment program (Torti et al., 1988).

The toxicity of this approach was quite acceptable, with essentially no bladder irritation and only mild interferon-induced flu symptoms. In addition to the acceptable toxicity profile of recombinant alpha-interon when delivered in this setting, a major advantage of this drug (over the use of BCG) is the availability of a standard treatment preparation for clinical use.

Recent experimental data have suggested that the activity of alpha-interferon against bladder tumor cell lines can be increased when the agent is encapsulated within liposomes (Killion et al., 1989). Clinical trials of the intravesical use of liposomal-encapsulated interferon would be of considerable interest.

5.4 Randomized clinical trials comparing various drugs for intravesical therapy

A number of randomized clinical trials have been conducted comparing different intravesical treatment approaches.

In a study at the Mayo Clinic, patients undergoing transurethral surgical resection of superficial bladder cancer were treated with thiotepa, doxorubicin, or placebo (Zincke et al., 1983). Whereas 71 percent of patients in the control group had recurrence of disease by 4 months postoperatively, 30 and 32 percent of patients receiving thiotepa and doxorubicin, respectively, had disease recurrence. There was no statistically significant difference between the two treatment options.

In a second trial from the same institution patients were randomized to receive either intravesical thiotepa or mitomycin C following surgical resection of superficial bladder cancer (Zincke et al., 1985). Again, there was no difference between the two treatment groups, with a 1-year recurrence rate of approximately 30 percent in each arm of the trial.

The National Bladder Cancer Group compared the clinical efficacy of intravesical thiotepa with that of mitomycin C in ablating residual superficial bladder cancer (Heney et al., 1988). The overall complete response rate with thiotepa was 26 percent compared with 39 percent for mitomycin C ($p = .08$). When partial responses were included, the total response rate for thiotepa was 53 percent and for mitomycin C 63 percent ($p = .23$). Bone marrow suppression was observed with both treatment programs, but rash was more common in patients receiving mitomycin C than in those treated with thiotepa.

Several trials have examined the clinical utility of intravesical BCG versus chemotherapy (Guinan, Crispen, and Rubenstein, 1987). In a small study (49 patients) reported from the University of California, Los Angeles, patients with superficial bladder cancer were randomized to receive either BCG (Tice strain) or thiotepa following surgical tumor removal (Brosman, 1982). At the time of the report (21-month mean follow-up), no recurrence had been found in the patients treated with BCG, whereas a 40 percent recurrence rate was found in patients randomized to thiotepa.

In a preliminary report of a large randomized trial (285 patients) comparing intravesical BCG (Connaught strain) with doxorubicin, recurrences were seen in 58 percent of the BCG-treated patients compared with 80 percent of the doxorubicin-treated patients (Lamm et al., 1989). In carcinoma in situ, 74 percent of patients treated with BCG achieved a complete response, compared with a 42 percent complete response rate in the patient population randomized to receive doxorubicin. In addition, the duration of the complete remission was considerably longer in those individuals achieving this clinical state following treatment with BCG. A recent review of a nonrandomized experience comparing BCG with doxorubicin supports the general conclusion that BCG is the superior agent, particularly in patients with incompletely resected tumors (Khanna, Son, et al., 1988).

An interim analysis of a randomized trial comparing the prophylactic intravesical administration of doxorubicin, thiotepa, or BCG in patients with superficial bladder cancer has demonstrated a statistically significant decrease in recurrence rate in the BCG-treated patients (9 of 67), compared with individuals treated with doxorubicin (23 of 53) or thiotepa (20 of 56) (Martinez-Pineiro et al., 1990).

It should be noted, however, that in a preliminary report of a randomized study comparing intravesical BCG with mitomycin C, no statistically significant difference in outcome (toxicity or efficacy) was observed (DeBruyne et al., 1988).

5.5 Summary and recommendations

Numerous trials have now solidly established the fact that intravesical therapy for superficial bladder cancer results in complete remissions in patients with residual disease and decreases the overall rate of tumor recurrence (Heney, 1988). It remains uncertain whether one particular chemotherapeutic or biologic agent is superior to any other. Of interest, an experimental model has suggested that the intravesical instillation of either doxorubicin or mitomycin C will actually promote bladder carcinogenesis

(Ohtani et al., 1984). At this time the clinical significance of these findings is unknown.

Recent data have suggested that BCG might be the agent of choice for intravesical therapy, particularly for carcinoma in situ of the bladder (Lamm et al., 1989). The recent approval by the U.S. Food and Drug Administration of a BCG preparation for intravesical delivery is an important development in the management of patients with superficial bladder cancer.

One final note of caution must be raised regarding the intravesical treatment of carcinoma in situ of the bladder. Although this therapeutic approach is reasonable and may avoid the need for cystectomy, evidence of persistent tumor following such treatment should lead to a more aggressive surgical approach, because continued conservative treatment may result in disease progression and death in a situation where surgery can be curative (Prout, Griffin, and Daly, 1987; Stanisic et al., 1987).

6 Intrathecal Therapy for Leukemia, Lymphoma, and Meningeal Carcinomatosis

6.1 Scope of the clinical problem

Involvement of the meninges by leukemia and lymphomas (particularly diffuse and undifferentiated histologies) has long been recognized to be an important clinical feature of these diseases (Aur et al., 1971; Bunn et al., 1976; Burchenal, 1983; Dawson, Rosenthal, and Maloney, 1973; Griffin et al., 1971; Haaxma-Reiche and Van Imhoff, 1989; Litam et al., 1979; Mackintosh et al., 1982; Price and Johnson, 1973; Sariban et al., 1983). For example, prior to the practice of administering central nervous system prophylaxis, more than 50 percent of children with acute lymphocytic leukemia developed central nervous system relapse after achieving a complete remission with systemic chemotherapy (Aur et al., 1971).

More recently, the importance of meningeal involvement as a site of metastatic spread has been recognized as a serious problem in patients with solid tumors, particularly small-cell lung cancer and carcinoma of the breast (Balducci et al., 1984; Nugent et al., 1979; Posner, 1977; Sculier, 1985; Sondak et al., 1981; Wasserstrom, Glass, and Posner, 1982; Yap et al., 1978). It has been suggested that the observed increased incidence of leptomeningeal carcinomatosis is the result of the success of systemic chemotherapy in prolonging survival and allowing time for neurologic complications of the disease to become clinically apparent (Posner, 1977; Sculier, 1985; Sondak et al., 1981). In addition, the concentration of most chemotherapeutic agents in the central nervous system following intravenous delivery is probably insufficient to produce a major cytotoxic effect (Shapiro, Young, and Mehta, 1975; Ushio, Posner, and Shapiro, 1977). Thus, the central nervous system serves as a sanctuary site for metastatic cancer.

The prognosis for patients found to have meningeal involvement with cancer varies considerably on the basis of the underlying malignancy and responsiveness to therapy. Patients with hematologic malignancies and central nervous system relapse may experience prolonged survival following both systemic and intrathecal drug delivery (Bleyer, 1984).

In contrast, in patients with solid tumors in whom treatment is far less successful, the median survival for treated patients may increase to 3 to 6 months compared with less than 2 months for untreated patients (Balducci et al., 1984; Giannone, Greco, and Hainsworth, 1986; Posner, 1977; Sause et al., 1988; Sculier, 1985; Sondak et al., 1981; Trump et al., 1982; Wasserstrom, Glass, and Posner, 1982). However, occasional patients with breast cancer and other malignancies may survive more than 1 to 2 years following regional drug delivery (lumbar intrathecal or intraventricular) and local radiation therapy (Levin et al., 1983; Sculier, 1985; Trump et al., 1982; Wasserstrom, Glass, and Posner, 1982; Yap et al., 1982). One report has noted that 25 percent of patients with leptomeningeal metastases from breast cancer will survive for more than 1 year following intraventricular therapy (with or without whole-brain radiotherapy) (Ongerboer De Visser et al., 1983). This relatively positive influence of therapy is far less likely in patients with meningeal involvement from lung cancer or melanoma (Posner, 1977; Wasserstrom, Glass, and Posner, 1982).

6.2 Rationale for regional drug delivery in the management of meningeal carcinomatosis

The administration of antineoplastic agents directly into the central nervous system, via either the lumbar intrathecal or the intraventricular route, has been demonstrated to markedly increase the concentration of the drug bathing the meninges compared with systemic drug delivery (Sculier, 1985; Shapiro, Young, and Mehta, 1975).

Unfortunately, as with other types of regional drug delivery, the depth of penetration of the cytotoxic drugs is limited to less than 1 to 2 mm from the meningeal surface (Blasberg, Patlak, and Fenstermacher, 1975). For this reason, external radiation therapy to any area of bulk disease (as demonstrated on myelogram) has been advocated by some investigators along with intrathecal drug administration for the diffuse microscopic disease present throughout the spinal fluid (Posner, 1977; Sculier, 1985; Wasserstrom, Glass, and Posner, 1982).

6.3 Regional therapy of meningeal carcinomatosis: lumbar intrathecal or intraventricular administration?

The question as to the superior local route for administering treatment to the meninges—intrathecal versus intraventricular—remains one of the more controversial issues in clinical oncology (Burchenal, 1983). Pharmacokinetic analysis supports an advantage for improved distribution of the drug within the spinal fluid following intraventricular as compared with lumbar intrathecal drug administration (Shapiro, Young, and Mehta, 1975). In the case of acute leukemia, limited clinical data support the superiority of this route of drug delivery in terms of a lower risk of development of recurrent meningeal leukemia (Bleyer and Poplack, 1979; Shapiro et al., 1977), although other investigators have come to the conclusion that the two routes of regional drug delivery produce comparable clinical results (Green et al., 1982; Haghbin and Galicich, 1979). In addition, the implanted reservoir device itself can be associated with significant morbidity, most notably the introduction of infection (Bleyer, Dizzo, et al., 1978; Dinndorf and Bleyer, 1987; Green et al., 1982; Lishner et al., 1990; Ommaya, 1984).

With meningeal carcinomatosis from solid tumors, most investigators have employed and recommended the intraventricular route of drug delivery (Giannone, Greco, and Hainsworth, 1986; Hitchins et al., 1987; Ongerboer De Visser et al., 1983; Trump et al., 1982; Wasserstrom, Glass, and Posner, 1982), although there are no trials that clearly prove the superiority of this approach (Posner, 1977). Several reasons have been advanced to support this method of administering antineoplastic drugs to the central nervous system.

First, as previously noted, pharmacokinetic evaluation has suggested that the distribution of drugs throughout the spinal fluid is superior with intraventricular delivery (Shapiro, Young, and Mehta, 1975). However, this may not be true when drugs that rapidly exit the spinal fluid (e.g., thiotepa) are administered by the intraventricular route (Strong et al., 1986). Under these conditions, drug levels in the lumbar spinal cerebrospinal fluid may only equal those found in the plasma and be far lower than that achieved in the ventricles.

Second, because therapy must be repeated weekly or twice a week, multiple lumbar punctures may be associated with considerable patient discomfort and potential morbidity. The surgical placement of an indwelling intraventricular catheter for the purpose of delivering treatment greatly facilitates treatment delivery (Ommaya, 1984; Wasserstrom, Glass, and Posner, 1982). In addition, percutaneous instillation of the drug into the lumbar spinal fluid frequently results in delivery of the agent into the epidural or subdural space rather than the subarachnoid space (Posner, 1977).

6.4 Selection of agents for regional therapy for meningeal carcinomatosis

One of the major limiting factors in developing an effective therapeutic program for meningeal carcinomatosis is the fact that very few drugs have been shown to have an acceptable toxicity profile when delivered directly into the subarachnoid space (Exhibit 6.1) (Bleyer, 1977).

Methotrexate is the agent most commonly employed when patients with either hematopoietic malignancies or solid tumors are treated by the lumbar intrathecal or intraventricular routes (Aur et al., 1971; Bleyer, 1984; Giannone, Greco, and Hainsworth, 1986; Haaxma-Reiche and Van Imhoff, 1989; Ongerboer De Visser et al., 1983; Posner, 1977; Shapiro et al., 1977; Trump et al., 1982; Wasserstrom, Glass, and Posner, 1982; Yap et al., 1982; Young et al., 1979). A number of intrathecal methotrexate treatment regimens have been employed. One of the most widely used approaches has been to initially administer the agent at a dose of 7 mg/m^2 twice a week (assuming an acceptable bone marrow status and renal function) until there is evidence of symptomatic improvement and clearing of malignant cells from the spinal fluid. The frequency of treatment is then reduced until the individual is being treated approximately once a month (maintenance phase) (Posner, 1977).

In patients with limited marrow reserve and to prevent methotrexate-induced stomatitis, the oral administration of folinic acid (10 mg orally twice a day for 3 days) beginning at least 12 hours after intrathecal methotrexate delivery has been shown to protect against the systemic side effects of the chemotherapeutic agent while not interfering with its cytotoxic effects

---

Exhibit 6.1

Antineoplastic Agents with Demonstrated Activity and Safety Following Intrathecal/Intraventricular Delivery

Methotrexate

Thiotepa

Cytarabine

against meningeal tumor (Mehta, Glass, and Shapiro, 1983; Sculier, 1985).

It is critical to remember that the methotrexate administered into the central nervous system *must* be preservative free.

Despite its relative safety, the intrathecal administration of methotrexate can be associated with serious morbidity and even mortality, especially when delivered with whole-brain radiotherapy (Bleyer, Drake, and Chabner, 1973; Clark et al., 1982; Duttera et al., 1973; Norrell et al., 1974; Peylan-Ramu et al., 1978; Posner, 1977). Systemic toxicities include bone marrow suppression, stomatitis, and even interstitial pneumonitis (Gutin, Green, et al., 1976).

Of greater concern, however, are the local side effects of this therapy, including chemical arachnoiditis and the development of a myelopathy (lower extremity pain, sensory loss, weakness, and paraplegia) or leukoencephalopathy (dementia, stupor, and seizures). Neuropathologic examination demonstrates multifocal necrosis, periventricular calcifications, acute fibrinoid changes in the blood vessels, and extensive vacuolar demyelination (Bates et al., 1985; Clark et al., 1982; Rubinstein et al., 1975).

In a rabbit model, investigators at Johns Hopkins University have demonstrated high levels of cytotoxic drugs in the substantia gelatinosa and peripheral white matter following intrathecal drug delivery, the same areas observed to be involved on histopathologic examination of the spinal column in individuals developing a myelopathy (Burch, Grossman, and Reinhard, 1988). In addition, extremely high levels of methotrexate in the cerebrospinal fluid following regional drug delivery have been observed to correlate with the subsequent development of neurotoxicity (Bleyer, Drake, and Chabner, 1973). The development of neurotoxic side effects secondary to abnormally high concentrations of drug in contact with the brain substance may be secondary to flow abnormalities preventing circulation and ultimate absorption of drug from the fluid (Grossman et al., 1982).

Various methods have been advocated to reduce the incidence and severity of toxicity associated with cytotoxic drug delivery into the central nervous system, including administering lower concentrations of the drug by longer infusions (Bleyer, Poplack, et al., 1978) and delivering the chemotherapeutic agent without radiation (Komp et al., 1982).

Other agents used for intrathecal administration as treatment of either hematologic malignancies or solid tumors involving the meninges include cytarabine (Band et al., 1973; Wang and Pratt, 1970), and thiotepa (Gutin et al., 1977; Gutin, Weiss, et al., 1976). Intrathecally delivered cytarabine has the added advantage of having a longer half-life in the spinal fluid than observed with systemic drug delivery (secondary to rapid deamination in the liver) of the agent (Burchenal, 1983). Toxicities similar to those seen with intrathecal methotrexate have been noted when either cytarabine or thiotepa is administered directly into the central nervous system (Breuer et al., 1977; Dunton et al., 1986; Gutin et al., 1977; Gutin, Weiss, et al., 1976). In the case of meningeal leukemia, single-agent cytarabine has been demonstrated to be active in patients failing intrathecal methotrexate (Band et al., 1973; Wang and Pratt, 1970).

Although combination intrathecal therapy has been employed (methotrexate and cytarabine; methotrexate and thiotepa; and methotrexate, thiotepa, and cytarabine), there is no evidence such therapy is superior to single-agent intrathecal treatment, and systemic toxicity will be increased (Giannone, Greco, and Hainsworth, 1986; Hitchins et al., 1987; Trump et al., 1982).

6.5 Summary and recommendations

To summarize the overall results of regional therapy of meningeal carcinomatosis, this therapeutic approach represents both the most and least successful efforts in regional antineoplastic drug delivery (Exhibit 6.2). Lumbar intrathecal or intraventricular therapy either as prophylaxis or therapy of known meningeal leukemia or lymphoma has contributed substantially to the improved outcomes currently anticipated for patients with these diseases.

Exhibit 6.2

Summary of the Status of Intrathecal/Intraventricular Antineoplastic Drug Delivery in the Management of Malignant Disease

---

Proven clinical benefit

    Prophylaxis of selected patients with leukemia/lymphoma

    Treatment of established meningeal leukemia/lymphoma

Possible clinical benefit

    Selected patients with meningeal carcinomatosis from breast cancer

Unproven or very limited clinical benefit

    Meningeal carcinomatosis from lung cancer or other solid tumors

Unfortunately, with the exception of 10 to 15 percent of patients with meningeal involvement from breast cancer, most patients with meningeal carcinomatosis from solid tumors will experience no, or only limited, benefit from regional antineoplastic drug delivery. It can reasonably be hoped that the development of new active cytotoxic agents that can be safely delivered into the subarachnoid space (Kooistra, Rodriguez, and Ponis, 1989; Laporte et al., 1985), unique methods of administration (e.g., cytarabine in liposomes [Hong and Mayhew, 1989; Kim et al., 1987]); or other innovative approaches, such as the delivery of intrathecal radiolabeled monoclonal antibodies with specificity for the tumor types involving the meninges (Lashford et al., 1988) or the use of regionally administered radiosensitizers with radiation therapy (Deutsch et al., 1989), will improve the outcome of treatment for individuals with meningeal carcinomatosis.

7 Development of a Model to Evaluate the Cost-Effectiveness of Regional versus Systemic Antineoplastic Therapy

In this chapter a method of evaluating the effectiveness of regional therapy relative to the costs is presented. In general, regional therapy is more expensive than standard systemically delivered chemotherapy. This is due to several factors: (a) Devices must be surgically or percutaneously placed to deliver treatment, (b) greater physician/nursing time and expertise are necessary, and (c) additional hospitalization may be essential to safely treat a patient by this therapeutic approach.

First, the difficulties in developing a reasonable model of cost versus effectiveness in clinical oncology are outlined and justification for the parameters included in this model is offered. This discussion is followed by an example of how the model might be used to evaluate the effectiveness of a specific regional chemotherapy technique in a particular disease setting. The example selected is hepatic artery infusion of chemotherapy for colon carcinoma metastatic to the liver. Data regarding the therapeutic efficacy of hepatic artery infusion versus systemic therapy are presented in detail in Chapter 2. An estimate of the costs associated with the two therapeutic approaches has been provided by Stagg et al. (1985).

7.1 Potential measures of effectiveness of cancer therapy

When discussing the effectiveness of a particular cancer therapy, a number of clinical end points might conceivably be used. These are described below.

7.1.1 Survival

There can be little question that the optimal end point to examine with any antineoplastic therapy is its impact on survival. Unfortunately, for several reasons this is often a difficult, if not possible, end point to analyze. First, in order to determine whether a particular therapy has had an impact on survival one must know the survival of a comparable untreated population or include a group of patients randomized to receive either no treatment or a "standard" therapeutic regimen (randomized controlled clinical trial). Defining appropriate comparative populations is often very difficult because of the heterogeneity in the extent of disease and patient performance status at the initiation of therapy. In addition, patient age and prior treatment history are often important clinical variables. Also, randomized trials are very expensive, usually require large numbers of patients, and may take years to complete.

Second, in patients who fail to respond to the treatment or who initially respond and then require alternative therapy, the impact of the specific treatment program under evaluation on overall survival may be difficult to define. For example, if no overall survival advantage is evident following the administration of a particular treatment, it might be that a response to second-line therapy has obscured the benefit. This is more than a theoretical concern because in randomized trials, for ethical reasons and as a strategy to ensure adequate patient accrual, a crossover design (to the alternative regimen) is frequently employed (Kemeny et al., 1987b). Thus, the "control" population may also receive the experimental treatment following failure of conventional therapy, and at the end of the trial no overall impact on survival may be observed even though one may truly exist.

If one chooses to use survival in an analysis of cost-effectiveness when cure is not a realistic goal (as is the situation with state-of-the-art therapy for most patients with advanced malignancies), it is necessary to define the survival end points to be used.

Median survival is a commonly reported end point in many clinical trials of therapy for advanced cancers. This would appear to be a reasonable measure of the benefit of treatment (keeping in mind the previously noted difficulties in comparing the results with those of other treatment options).

However, it is proposed in this model that along with median survival a second end point be included. This survival time point is the longer survival of a minority of the treated population (tail of the survival curve). As a society we have been willing to pay for therapies that produce a significant benefit for a relatively small patient population (Markman, 1988). Although it is not appropriate to suggest that large sums should be spent to benefit only 1 or 2 percent of patients treated with a therapeutic modality, a treatment resulting in prolonged survival for a somewhat larger subset of patients would probably be supported by our society.

Thus, for the purposes of this exercise, the 10 percent survival point is used as that "reasonable" subset of patients whose survival is included in this evaluation of cost versus effectiveness. (Readers may choose to select an alternative point to include in a modification of the present model.)

It is necessary to give a reasonable weight to the benefits associated with the survival of 10 percent of patients treated by a particular therapeutic approach compared with the survival of the remainder of the patient population. Because this subset of individuals represents one-fifth the median (50 percent survival), the added survival benefit assigned in the model to this group of patients is one-fifth (multiplied by 0.2) the weight given to the median survival.

7.1.2 Objective response rates

An alternative end point that has commonly been used by the oncology community to "suggest" the relative efficacy of a therapeutic approach is the objective response rate to treatment. Whereas studies performed in the 1960s and 1970s often failed to use standardized measures of response (making it impossible to compare one report with another), oncologists currently engaged in clinical research use very similar definitions of response to therapy within a particular disease category (Miller et al., 1981). In patient populations with similar clinical characteristics (as previously noted), objective response rates determined by different investigators will usually fall within reasonably comparable ranges (Kemeny, 1987; Markman, 1986).

Unfortunately, it is not always clear that a "response to therapy," particularly anything short of a complete response, will affect survival (Oye and Shapiro, 1984). For example, shrinkage of a tumor by 50 percent (standardly required for a patient to be considered to have experienced a partial response) may or may not result in an improvement in survival, depending on how long the response lasts, where the disease ultimately progresses, and how rapidly the tumor grows once the response ends. In addition, a 50 percent reduction in the size of a large mass may be quite different from a similar percent shrinkage of a very small tumor. Finally, the impact of such therapy on symptoms is often not clearly defined or quantified in reports suggesting a therapeutic benefit of treatment based solely on an improvement in response rate compared with a historical or even a randomized control population.

Despite these limitations, it is generally recognized that objective response rates are often the most quantifiable measures available for comparisons of the relative efficacies of cancer therapy. In addition, major antitumor responses are usually associated with a reduction in symptoms if any were present at the initiation of therapy.

Recognizing that all responding patients do not benefit with an improvement in survival or symptoms, and that even nonresponding patients live a finite period of time (either with no therapy or with symptomatic treatment only), the value of a response must be weighed in a reasonable manner relative to survival. In this model the response rate (percent response) is multiplied by the median survival to obtain a measure of its influence on cost versus effectiveness.

7.1.3 Quality of life

A positive impact on the quality of life of a patient with cancer is an alternative end point that has been suggested as a surrogate for improvement in survival (Aaronson, 1988; Goodwin et al., 1988; Schipper et al., 1984). Unfortunately, measures of quality of life, including an improvement in such symptoms as pain, are quite subjective and have yet to be shown to provide reproducible and clinically valid information upon which evaluations of therapeutic efficacy can be based (Donovan, Sanson-Fisher, and Redman, 1989; Ganz et al., 1988).

In addition, the perceptions of the patient and his or her family of the patient's quality of life are often quite different from that of the physician or other less biased observers (Danis et al., 1988). This fact makes it difficult to assume that individuals treated with experimental agents can provide an objective assessment of the positive or negative effects of a treatment on overall quality of life or even its impact on a specific symptom. The well-recognized placebo effect and the overwhelming desire on the part of the patient and his or her family to believe in the benefits of treatment of a potentially fatal disease make subjective evaluations suspect as measures of clinical effectiveness.

Finally, if quality of life measures are to have any meaning in assessing the efficacy of therapy, it is important to reevaluate the measurements every time there is a modification in a treatment protocol (changing to a weekly from a monthly schedule, increasing or decreasing the dose of a toxic agent by 20 percent, or adding or subtracting an agent from a regimen). This will add substantially to the cost of each trial and it is unlikely that the manpower required to properly conduct such as evaluation will be available for the numerous trials conducted in the United States and internationally.

Exhibit 7.1

Equation for Cost/Response–Survival Months

$$\frac{\text{Cost of therapy}}{\text{Med Surv} + (0.2)(10\% \text{ Surv}) + (\% \text{ Response}) (\text{Med Surv})}$$

where

Med Surv = median survival (in months),

10% = survival of longest surviving 10 percent of treated patients in months,

% Response = percentage of patients demonstrating at least a partial response.

7.2 Evaluation of cost versus effectiveness

In summary, any single measure of efficacy of antineoplastic therapy that might currently be employed in a cost-effectiveness analysis can be criticized for a number of reasons. Therefore, in the present model (Exhibit 7.1), three measures of effectiveness (median survival, 10 percent survival, and objective response rate) are used to decrease the risk that any policy decision based on such an analysis will fail to take into consideration the multiple compounding variables that make a reliable assessment of effectiveness of antineoplastic therapy difficult.

Solving the equation for a particular therapeutic approach gives a figure that shall be called the *cost per response–survival month* (Cost/R–S Month).

7.3 The cost per response–survival month for hepatic artery versus systemic chemotherapy for colon cancer metastatic to the liver

The standard (conventional) treatment of colon carcinoma metastatic to the liver is the systemic delivery of single-agent 5-FU or a 5-FU-based combination regimen (Kemeny, 1987). This therapy is generally delivered in the ambulatory setting. The response rate to such therapy is approximately 20 percent, with a median survival of 10 months. Ten percent of patients will survive 17 months from the initiation of therapy (Kemeny, 1987).

As previously discussed, hepatic arterial therapy can be delivered either by percutaneous catherization with each treatment course or by surgically

Table 7.1

**Sample Calculation of Cost/Response–Survival Months
for Hepatic Arterial Chemotherapy versus Systemic Therapy
for Colon Carcinoma Metastatic to the Liver**

	Intravenous chemotherapy	Hepatic arterial chemotherapy
Cost[a]	$6,500[b]	$15,500[b]
Median survival	10 mos.	18 mos.
10% survival	17 mos.	26 mos.
Response rate	20%	50%
Cost/Response– Survival Month	$6,500/(10 + (0.2)(17) + (0.20)(10)) = $422	$15,500/(18 + (0.2)(26) + (0.5)(18)) = $482

[a] For 8 months of therapy.
[b] Cost figures are from Stagg et al. (1985).

placing an implantable catheter attached to an infusion pump. Because the surgically implanted approach is more often used in the community, this shall be employed in the present example.

Costs of hepatic arterial therapy not generally encountered with systemic treatment include surgical fees, operating room time, the device/catheter, radiology charges, charges for frequent visits to "load" the port with chemotherapy or to administer drugs to prevent the catheter from clotting, and added hospitalizations for drug administration (principally with the percutaneous devices) and complications of the catheters (principally infection) (Stagg et al., 1985). The response rate to hepatic arterial therapy in colon carcinoma metastatic to the liver is approximately 50 percent, with a median survival of 18 months (Kemeny et al., 1987; Venook, Stagg, and Lewis, 1988). Approximately 10 percent of patients will survive 26 months following the initiation of this therapeutic approach (Kemeny et al., 1987).

Table 7.1 summarizes the data presented in the preceding paragraph and demonstrates the calculation of the Cost/R–S Month for both hepatic artery and systemic therapy. Comparison of the absolute values of these two numbers has limited meaning because the figures do not reflect actual resources used. Rather, the percent increase in cost of the alternative (and less costly) strategy should be examined relative to the objective benefits of the more expensive treatment.

It is suggested from the perspective of the health policy analyst that in the present example, an increase in the Cost/R–S Month ratio of 14 percent—($482 − $422) / $422—would appear to be a reasonable expenditure of resources when the benefits of hepatic arterial therapy (symptom relief and possible prolongation of survival) are considered.

This model, with or without modifications, can be employed to compare other forms of regional therapy (or other investigative approaches) with standard systemic treatment strategies.

References

Aaronson, N. K. (1988) Quality of life: What is it? How should it be measured? *Oncology* 2(5):69–74.

Abe, R., Akiyoshi, T., Koba, F., Tsuji, H., & Baba, T. (1988) 'Two-route chemotherapy' using intra-arterial cisplatin and intravenous sodium thiosulfate, its neutralizing agent, for hepatic malignancies. *Eur J Cancer Clin Oncol* 24:1671–1674.

Ackerman, N. B. (1974) The blood supply of experimental liver metastases. IV. Changes in vascularity with increasing tumor growth. *Surgery* 75:589–596.

Ackerman, N. B. (1986) Experimental studies on the role of the portal circulation in hepatic tumor vascularity. *Cancer* 58:1653–1657.

Ackerman, D., Biedermann, C., Bailly, G., & Studer, U. E. (1988) Treatment of superficial bladder tumors with intravesical recombinant interferon alpha-2a. *Urol Int* 43(2):85–88.

Adams, S. C., Patt, Y. Z., & Rosenblum, M. G. (1984) Pharmacokinetics of mitomycin c following intraperitoneal administration of mitomycin c and floxuridine for peritoneal carcinomatosis (abstract). *Proc Am Assoc Cancer Res* 25:361.

Adson, M. A. & Van Heerden, J. A. (1980) Major hepatic resections for metastatic colorectal cancer. *Ann Surg* 191:576–583.

Aigner, K. R. (1988) Isolated liver perfusion: 5-year results. *Reg Cancer Treat* 1:11–20.

Aigner, K., Hild, P., Henneking, K., Paul, E., & Hundeiker, M. (1983) Regional perfusion with cis-platinum and decarbazine. *Recent Results Cancer Res* 86:239–245.

Aigner, K. R., Walther, H., Muller, H., Jansa, J., & Thiem, N. (1988) Intra-arterial infusion chemotherapy for recurrent breast cancer. *Reg Cancer Treat* 1:102–107.

Aisner, J., & Wiernik, P. H. (1981) Chemotherapy in the treatment of malignant mesothelioma. *Semin Oncol* 8:335–343.

Ajani, J. A., Carrasco, C. H., Jackson, D. E., & Wallace, S. (1989) Combination of cisplatin plus fluoropyrimidine chemotherapy effective against liver metastases from carcinoma of the anal canal. *Am J Med* 87:221–224.

Albano, W. A., Durr, M., Gutierrez, A. R., McGill, J., Campbell, A., Mailliard, J. A., Johnson, P. S., Dvorak, A. D., Lynch, H. T., & Fitzgibbons, R. J., Jr. (1984) Hepatic artery infusion: Surgical approach. *Cancer Drug Deliv* 1:213–226.

Alberts, A. S., Falkson, G., Goedhals, L., Vorobiof, D. A., & Van Der Merve, C. A.

(1988) Malignant pleural mesothelioma: A disease unaffected by current therapeutic maneuvers. *J Clin Oncol* 6:527–535.

Alberts, D. S., Chen, H. S. G., Chang, S. Y., & Peng, Y. M. (1980) The disposition of intraperitoneal bleomycin, melphalan, and vinblastine in cancer patients. *Recent Results Cancer Res* 74:293–299.

Alberts, D. S., Chen, H. S. G., Mayersohn, M., Perrier, D., Moon, T. E., & Gross, J. F. (1979) Bleomycin pharmacokinetics in man. II. Intracavitary administration. *Cancer Chemother Pharmacol* 2:127–132.

Alberts, D. S., Hilgers, R. D., Moon, T. E., Martimbeau, P. W., & Rivkin, S. (1979) Combination chemotherapy for alkylator-resistant ovarian carcinoma: A preliminary report of a Southwest Oncology Group trial. *Cancer Treat Rep* 63:301–305.

Alberts, D. S., Peng, Y-M., Leigh, S., Davis, T. P., & Woodward, D. L. (1985) Disposition of mitoxantrone in cancer patients. *Cancer Res* 45:1879–1884.

Alberts, D. S., Surwit, E. A., Peng, Y-M., McCloskey, T., Rivest, R., Graham, V., McDonald, L., & Roe, D. (1988) Phase I clinical and pharmacokinetic study of mitoxantrone given to patients by intraperitoneal administration. *Cancer Res* 48:5874–5877.

Alberts, D. S., Young, L., Mason, N., & Salmon, S. E. (1985) In vitro evaluation of anticancer drugs against ovarian cancer at concentrations achievable by intraperitoneal administration. *Semin Oncol* 12(3; Suppl. 4):38–42.

Allen, L. M., Tejada, F., Okonmah, A. D., & Nordqvist, S. (1982) Combination chemotherapy of the epipodophyllotoxin derivatives, teniposide and etoposide: A pharmacodynamic rationale? *Cancer Chemother Pharmacol* 7:151–156.

Andrews, P. A., Velury, S., Mann, S. C., & Howell, S. B. (1988) Cis-diamminedichloroplatinum(II) accumulation in sensitive and resistant human ovarian carcinoma cells. *Cancer Res* 48:68–73.

Ansfield, F. J., & Ramirez, G. (1978) The clinical results of 5-fluorouracil intrahepatic arterial infusion in 528 patients with metastatic cancer to the liver. *Prog Clin Cancer* 7:201–206.

Antman, K. H. (1981) Clinical presentation and natural history of benign and malignant mesothelioma. *Semin Oncol* 8:313–320.

Antman, K. H., Klegar, K. L., Pomfret, E. A., Osteen, R. T., Amato, D. A., Larson, D. A., & Corson, J. M. (1985) Early peritoneal mesothelioma: A treatable malignancy. *Lancet* 2:977–980.

Antman, K., Shemin, R., Ryan, L., Klegar, K., Osteen, R., Herman, T., Lederman, G., & Corson, J. (1988) Malignant mesothelioma: Prognostic variables in a registry of 180 patients, the Dana-Farber Cancer Institute and Brigham and Women's Hospital experience over two decades. 1965–1985. *J Clin Oncol* 6:147–153.

Arbuck, S. G., Trave, F., Douglass, H. O., Jr., Nava, H., Zakrzewski, S., & Rustum, Y. M. (1986) Phase 1 and pharmacologic studies of intraperitoneal leucovorin and 5-fluorouracil in patients with advanced cancer. *J Clin Oncol* 4:1510–1517.

Archer, S. G., McCulloch, R. K., & Gray, B. N. (1989) A comparative study of the pharmacokinetics of continuous portal vein infusion versus intraperitoneal infusion of 5-fluorouracil. *Reg Cancer Treat* 2:105–111.

Ariel, I. M., Oropeza, R., & Pack, G. T. (1966) Intracavitary administration of radioactive isotopes in the control of effusions due to cancer: Results in 267 patients. *Cancer* 19:1096–1102.

August, D. A., Sugarbaker, P. H., Ottow, R. T., Gianola, F. J., & Schneider, P. D. (1985) Hepatic resection of colorectal metastases: Influence of clinical factors and adjuvant intraperitoneal 5-fluorouracil via Teckhoff catheter on survival. *Ann Surg* 201:210–218.

Aur, R. J. A., Simone, J., Hustu, H. O., Walters, T., Borella, L., Pratt, C., & Pinkel, D. (1971) Central nervous system therapy and combination chemotherapy of childhood lymphocytic leukemia. *Blood* 37:272–281.

Austin, E. H., & Flye, M. W. (1979) The treatment of recurrent malignant pleural effusion. *Ann Thorac Surg* 28:190–203.

Azzarelli, A., Gennari, L., Bonfanti, G., Audisio, R., & Quagliuolo, V. (1983) Intraarterial adriamycin for limb sarcomas. *Recent Results Cancer Res* 86:218–222.

Baas, P. C., Hoekstra, H. J., Koops, H. S., Oosterhuis, W. J., & Van Der Weele, L. T. (1989) Hyperthermic isolated regional perfusion in the treatment of extremity melanoma in children and adolescents. *Cancer* 63:199–203.

Baas, P. C., Koops, H. S., Hoekstra, H. J., Oosterhuis, J. W., van der Welle, L. T., & Oldhoff, J. (1988) Isolated regional perfusion in the treatment of local recurrence, satellitosis and in-transit metastases of melanomas of the extremities. *Reg Cancer Treat* 1:22–36.

Badalament, R. A., Gay, H., Cibas, E. S., Herr, H. W., Whitmore, W. F., Jr., Fair, W. R., & Melamed, M. R. (1987) Monitoring intravesical Bacillus Calmette-Guerin treatment of superficial bladder carcinoma by postoperative urinary cytology. *J Urol* 138:763–765.

Bajorin, D., Kelsen, D., & Mintzer, D. M. (1987) Phase II trial of mitomycin in malignant mesothelioma. *Cancer Treat Rep* 71:857–858.

Baker, S. R., & Wheeler, R. H. (1982) Long-term intraarterial chemotherapy infusion of ambulatory head and neck cancer patients. *J Surg Oncol* 21:125–131.

Baker, S. R., & Wheeler, R. H. (1984) Intraarterial chemotherapy for head and neck cancer, part 2: Clinical experience. *Head Neck Surg* 6:751–760.

Baker, S. R., Wheeler, R. H., Ensminger, W. D., & Nieederhuber, J. E. (1981) Intraarterial infusion chemotherapy for head and neck cancer using a totally implantable infusion pump. *Head Neck Surg* 4:118–124.

Baker, S. R., Wheeler, R. H., Ziessman, H. A., Medvec, B. R., Thrall, J. H., & Keyes, J. W., Jr. (1984) Radionuclide localization of intraarterial infusions in head and neck cancer. *Cancer Drug Deliv* 1(2):145–156.

Balch, C. M., Urist, M. M., Soong, S-J., & McGregor, M. (1983) A prospective phase II clinical trial of continuous FUDR regional chemotherapy for colorectal metastases to the liver using a totally implantable drug infusion pump. *Ann Surg* 198:567–573.

Balducci, L., Little, D. D., Khansur, T., & Steinberg, M. H. (1984) Carcinomatous meningitis in small cell lung cancer. *Am J Med Sci* 287:31–33.

Band, P. R., Holland, J. F., Bernard, J., Weil, M., Walker, M., & Rall, D. (1973) Treatment of central nervous system leukemia with intrathecal cytosine arabinoside. *Cancer* 32:744–748.

Banks, M. D., Pontes, J. E., Izbicki, R. M., & Pierce, J. M., Jr. (1977) Topical instillation of doxorubicin hydrochloride in the treatment of recurring superficial transitional cell carcinoma of the bladder. *J Urol* 118:757–760.

Barone, R. M. (1986) Indication and rationale for the use of implantable devices for arterial regional chemotherapy. *Recent Results Cancer Res* 100:163–170.

Bast, R. C., Berek, J. S., Obrist, R., Griffiths, C. T., Berkowitz, R. S., Hacker, N. F., Parker, L., Lagasse, L. D., & Knapp, R. C. (1983) Intraperitoneal immunotherapy of human ovarian carcinoma with *Corynebacterium parvum. Cancer Res* 43:1395–1401.

Bates, S., McKeever, P., Masur, H., Levens, D., Macher, A., Armstrong, G., & Magrath, I. T. (1985) Myelopathy following intrathecal chemotherapy in a patient with extensive Burkitt's lymphoma and altered immune status. *Am J Med* 78:697–702.

Batist, G., Ihde, D. C., Zabell, A., Lichter, A. S., Veach, S. R., Cohen, M. H., Carney, D. N., & Bunn, P. A. (1983) Small-cell carcinoma of the lung: Reinduction therapy after late relapse. *Ann Intern Med* 98:472–474.

Bedikian, A. Y. (1983) Regional and systemic chemotherapy for advanced colorectal cancer: A review. *Dis Colon Rectum* 26:327–332.

Bedikian, A. Y., Chen, T. T., Malahy, M-A., Patt, Y. Z., & Bodey, G. P. (1984) Prognostic factors influencing survival of patients with advanced colorectal cancer: Hepatic-artery infusion versus systemic intravenous chemotherapy for liver metastases. *J Clin Oncol* 2:174–180.

Beller, U., Chachoua, A., Speyer, J. L., Sorich, J., Dugan, M., Liebes, L., Hayes, R., & Beckman, E. M. (1989) Phase 1B study of low-dose intraperitoneal recombinant interleukin-2 in patients with refractory advanced ovarian cancer: Rationale and preliminary report. *Gynecol Oncol* 34:407–412.

Bengtsson, G., Carlsson, G., Hafstrom, L., & Jonsson, R-E. (1981) Natural history of patients with untreated liver metastases from colorectal cancer. *Am J Surg* 141:586–589.

Benjamin, R. S. (1989) Regional chemotherapy for osteosarcoma. *Semin Oncol* 16:323–327.

Berek, J. S., Hacker, N. F., Lichtenstein, A., Jung, T., Spina, C., Knox, R. M., Brady, J., Greene, T., Ettinger, L. M., Lagasse, L., Bonnem, E. M., Spiegel, R. J., & Zighelboim, J. (1985) Intraperitoneal recombinant alpha-interferon for "salvage" immunotherapy in stage III epithelial ovarian cancer: A Gynecologic Oncology Group study. *Cancer Res* 45:4447–4453.

Berek, J., Knapp, R., Hacker, N., Lichtenstein, A., Jung, T., Spina, C., Obrist, R., Griffiths, C. T., Berkowitz, R. S., Parker, L., Zighelboim, J., & Bast, R. C. (1985) Intraperitoneal immunotherapy of human ovarian carcinoma with *Corynebacterium parvum. Am J Obstet Gynecol* 152:1003–1010.

Bergman, F. (1966) Carcinoma of the ovary: A clinicopathological study of 86 autopsied cases with special reference to mode of spread. *Acta Obstet Gynecol Scand* 45:211–231.

Bertelsen, K., Jakobsen, A., Kern, M., Hansen, G., Larsen, M., Nylan, M., Panduro, J., Pedersen, P. H., Stroyer, I., & Andersen, J. E. (1989) A randomized trial of six cycles versus twelve cycles of cycloiphosphamide, adriamycin and cis-platinum in advanced ovarian cancer (abstract). *Proc Am Soc Clin Oncol* 8:150.

Bezwoda, W. R., Seymour, L., & Dansey, R. (1989) Intraperitoneal recombinant interferon-alpha 2b for recurrent malignant ascites due to ovarian cancer. *Cancer* 64:1029–1033.

Bierman, H. R., Byron, R. L., Kelley, K. H., & Grady, A. (1951) Studies on the blood supply of tumor in man. III. Vascular patterns of the liver by hepatic arteriography in vivo. *JNCI* 12:107–111.

Bitran, J. D. (1985) Intraperitoneal bleomycin, pharmacokinetics and results of a phase 2 trial. *Cancer* 56:2420–2423.

Bitran, J. D., Brown, C., Desser, R. K., Kozloff, M. F., Shapiro, C., & Billings, A. A. (1981) Intracavitary bleomycin for the control of malignant effusions. *J Surg Oncol* 16:273–277.

Blackledge, G., Lawton, F., Buckley, H., & Crowther, D. (1984) Phase II evaluation of bleomycin in patients with advanced epithelial ovarian cancer. *Cancer Treat Rep* 68:549–550.

Bland, K. I., Kimura, A. K., Brenner, D. E., Basinger, M. A., Hirsch, M., Hawkins, I. F., Pierson, K. K., & Copeland, E. M., III. (1989) A phase II study of the efficacy of diamminedichloroplatinum (cisplatin) for the control of locally recurrent and intransit malignant melanoma of the extremities using tourniquet outflow-occlusion techniques. *Ann Surg* 209:73–80.

Blasberg, R. G., Patlak, C., & Fenstermacher, J. D. (1975) Intrathecal chemotherapy: Brain tissue profiles after ventriculo-cisternal perfusion. *J Pharmacol Exp Ther* 195:73–83.

Bleyer, W. A. (1977) Current status of intrathecal chemotherapy for human meningeal neoplasms. *Natl Cancer Inst Monogr* 46:171–178.

Bleyer, W. A. (1984) Intrathecal methotrexate versus central nervous system leukemia. *Cancer Drug Deliv* 1:157–167.

Bleyer, W. A., Drake, J. C., & Chabner, B. A. (1973) Neurotoxicity and elevated cerebrospinal-fluid methotrexate concentration in meningeal leukemia. *N Engl J Med* 289:770–773.

Bleyer, W. A., Pizzo, P. A., Spence, A. M., Platt, W. D., Benjamin, D. R., Kolins, J., & Poplack, D. G. (1978) The Ommaya reservoir: Newly recognized complications and recommendations for insertion and use. *Cancer* 41:2431–2437.

Bleyer, W. A., & Poplack, D. G. (1979) Intraventricular versus intralumbar methotrexate for central-nervous-system leukemia: Prolonged remission with the Ommaya reservoir. *Med Pediatr Oncol* 6:207–213.

Bleyer, W. A., Poplack, D. G., Simon, R. M., Henderson, E. S., Leventhal, B. G., Zeigler, J. L., & Ommaya, A. K. (1978) "Concentration × time" methotrexate via a subcutaneous reservoir: A less toxic regimen for intraventricular chemotherapy of central nervous system neoplasms. *Blood* 51:835–842.

Blochl-Daum, B., Eichler, H. G., Rainer, H., Jakesz, R., Salzer, H., Steger, G., Schuller, J., Gunther, E., Proksch, P., & Ehninger, G. (1987) Phase I study of intraperitoneal mitoxantrone—clinical and pharmacokinetic evaluation. *Onkologie* 10(1):54–56.

Blochl-Daum, B., Eichler, H. G., Rainer, H., Jakesz, R., Salzer, H., Steger, G., Schuller, J., Gunther, E., Proksch, B., & Ehninger, G. (1988) Escalating dose regimen of intraperitoneal mitoxantrone: Phase I study—clinical and pharmacokinetic evaluation. *Eur J Cancer Clin Oncol* 24:1133–1138.

Blumenreich, M. S., Needles, B., Yagoda, A., Sogani, P., Grabstald, H., & Whitmore, W. F., Jr. (1982) Intravesical cisplatin for superficial bladder tumors. *Cancer* 50:863–865.

Boos, G., Thirlwell, M., Blanchard, R., Herba, M., Gonzalez, L., Rosenthall, L., Skelton, J., & Boileau, G. (1989) Phase I–II study of hepatic arterial infusion of yttrium-90 glass microspheres in cancer of the liver (abstract). *Proc Am Soc Clin Oncol* 8:103.

Bracken, R. B., Johnson, D. E., Swanson, D. A., De Furia, D., & Crooke, S. (1980) Role of intravesical mitomycin C in management of superficial bladder tumors. *Urology* 16:11–15.

Braly, P., Doroshow, J., & Hoff, S. (1986) Technical aspects of intraperitoneal chemotherapy in abdominal carcinomatosis. *Gynecol Oncol* 25:319–333.

Breedis, C., & Young, G. (1954) The blood supply of neoplasms in the liver. *Am J Pathol* 30:969–977.

Bretton, P. R., Herr, H. W., Kimmel, M., Fair, W. R., Whitmore, W. F., & Melamed, M. R. (1989) Flow cytometry as a predictor of response and progression in patients with superficial bladder cancer treated with Bacillus Calmette-Guerin. *J Urol* 141:1332–1336.

Bretton, P. R., Herr, H. W., Kimmel, M., Whitmore, W. F., Laudone, V., Oettgen, H. F., & Fair, W. F. (1990) The response of patients with superficial bladder cancer to a second course of intravesical Bacillus Calmette-Guerin. *J Urol* 143:710–713.

Breuer, A. C., Pitman, S. W., Dawson, D. M., & Schoene, W. E. (1977) Paraparesis following intrathecal cytosine arabinoside: A case report with neuropathologic findings. *Cancer* 40:2817–2822.

Briele, H. A., Djuric, M., Jung, D. T., Mortell, T., Patel, M. K., & Das Gupta, T. K. (1985) Pharmacokinetics of melphalan in clinical isolation perfusion of the extremities. *Cancer Res* 45:1885–1889.

Brosman, S. A. (1982) Experience with Bacillus Calmette-Guerin in patients with superficial bladder carcinoma. *J Urol* 128:27–30.

Brosman, S. A. (1985) The use of Bacillus Calmette-Guerin in the therapy of bladder carcinoma in situ. *J Urol* 134:36–39.

Bruckner, H. W., Wallach, R., Cohen, C. J., Deppe, G., Kabakow, B., Ratner, L., & Holland, J. F. (1981) High-dose platinum for the treatment of refractory ovarian cancer. *Gynecol Oncol* 12:64–67.

Buchwald, H., Grage, T. B., Vassilopoulos, P. P., Rohde, T. D., Varco, R. L., & Blackshear, P. J. (1980) Intraarterial infusion chemotherapy for hepatic carcinoma using a totally implantable infusion pump. *Cancer* 45:866–869.

Budd, G. T., Schreiber, M. J., Steiger, E., Bukowski, R. M., & Weick, J. K. (1986) Phase 1 trial of intraperitoneal chemotherapy with 5-fluorouracil and citrovorum factor. *Invest New Drugs* 4:155–158.

Bunn, P. A., Schein, P. S., Banks, P. M., & DeVita, V. T., Jr. (1976) Central nervous system complications in patients with diffuse histiocytic and undifferentiated lymphoma: Leukemia revisited. *Blood* 47:3–10.

Burch, P. A., Grossman, S. A., & Reinhard, C. S. (1988) Spinal cord penetration of intrathecally administered cytarabine and methotrexate: A quantitative autoradiographic study. *JNCI* 80:1211–1216.

Burchenal, J. H. (1983) History of intrathecal prophylaxis and therapy of meningeal leukemia. *Cancer Drug Deliv* 1:87–92.

Buroker, T., Samson, M., Correa, J., Fraile, R., & Vaitkevicius, V. K. (1976) Hepatic artery infusion of 5-FUDR after prior systemic 5-fluorouracil. *Cancer Treat Rep* 60:1277–1279.

Busse, O., Aigner, K., & Wilimzig, H. (1983) Peripheral nerve damage following isolated extremity perfusion with cis-platinum. *Recent Results Cancer Res* 86:264–267.

Cady, B., & Oberfield, R. A. (1974) Regional infusion chemotherapy of hepatic metastases from carcinoma of the colon. *Am J Surg* 127:220–227.

Cain, J. M., Saigo, P. E., Pierce, V. K., Clark, D. G., Jones, W. B., Smith, D. H., Hakes, T. B., Ochoa, M., & Lewis, J. L. (1986) A review of second-look laparotomy for ovarian cancer. *Gynecol Oncol* 23:14–25.

Calvo, D. B., Patt, Y. Z., Wallace, S., Chuang, V. P., Benjamin, R. S., Pritchard, J. D., Hersh, E. M., Bodey, G. P., & Mavligit, G. M. (1980) Phase I–II trial of percutaneous intra-arterial cis-diamminedichloroplatinum (II) for regionally confined malignancy. *Cancer* 45:1278–1283.

Camaggi, C. M., Strocchi, E., Costanti, B., Beghelli, P., Ferrari, P., & Pannuti, F. (1985) Medroxyprogesterone acetate bioavailability after high-dose intraperitoneal administration in advanced cancer. *Chemother Pharmacol* 14:232–234.

Canal, P., Bugat, R., Chatelut, E., Pinel, M. C., Houin, G., Plusquellec, Y., & Carton, M. (1989) Phase 1/pharmacokinetic study of intraperitoneal teniposide (VM 26). *Eur J Cancer Clin Oncol* 25(5):815–820.

Carlson, J. A., Jr., Litterst, C. L., Grenberg, R. A., Day, T. G., Jr., & Masterson, B. J. (1984) Platinum tissue concentrations following intra-arterial and intravenous cis-diamminedichloroplatinum II in New Zealand white rabbits. *Am J Obstet Gynecol* 148:313–317.

Carter, R. D., Faddis, D. M., Krementz, E. T., Salwen, W. A., Puyau, F. A., & Muchmore J. H. (1988) Treatment of locally advanced breast cancer with regional intra-arterial chemotherapy. *Reg Cancer Treat* 1:108–111.

Carter, S. K. (1977) The chemotherapy of head and neck cancer. *Semin Oncol* 4:413–424.

Cascino, T. L., Byrne, T. N., Deck, M. D. F., & Posner, J. B. (1983) Intra-arterial BCNU in the treatment of metastatic brain tumors. *J Neurol Oncol* 1:211–218.

Casper, E. S., Kelsen, D. P., Alcock, N. W., & Lewis, J. L. (1983) Ip cisplatin in patients with malignant ascites: Pharmacokinetics evaluation and comparison with the iv route. *Cancer Treat Rep* 67:325–238.

Catalona, W. J., Hudson, M. A., Gillen, D. P., Andriole, G. L., & Ratliff, T. L. (1987) Risks and benefits of repeated courses of intravesical Bacillus Calmette-Guerin therapy for superficial bladder cancer. *J Urol* 137:220–224.

Chabner, B. A., Myers, C. E., Coleman, C. N., & Johns, D. G. (1975) The clinical pharmacology of antineoplastic agents. *N Engl J Med* 292:1107–1113.

Chahinian, A. P., Norton, L., Holland, J. F., Szrajer, L., & Hart, R. D. (1984) Experimental and clinical activity of mitomycin C and cis-diamminedichloroplatinum in malignant mesothelioma. *Cancer Res* 44:1688–1692.

Chambers, S. K., Chambers, J. T., Kohorn, E. I., & Schwartz, P. E. (1987) Etoposide (VP-16-213) plus cis-diamminedichloroplatinum as salvage therapy in advanced epithelial ovarian cancer. *Gynecol Oncol* 27:233–240.

Chan, C. K., Coppoc, G. L., Zimm, S., Cleary, S., & Howell, S. B. (1988) Pharmacokinetics of intraperitoneally administered dipyridamole in cancer patients. *Cancer Res* 48:215–218.

Chang, A. E., Collins, J. M., Speth, P. A. J., Smith, R., Rowland, J. B., Walton, L., Begley, M. G., Glatstein, E., & Kinsella, T. J. (1989) A phase 1 study of intra-arterial iododeoxyuridine in patients with colorectal liver metastases. *J Clin Oncol* 7:662–668.

Chang, A. E., Schneider, P. D., Sugarbaker, P. H., Simpson, C., Culnane, M., & Steinberg, S. M. (1987) A prospective randomized trial of regional versus systemic continuous 5-fluorodeoxyuridine chemotherapy of colorectal liver metastases. *Ann Surg* 206:685–693.

Chapman, P. B., Kolitz, J. E., Hakes, T., Gabrilove, J. L., Kolitz, J. E., Welte, K., Merluzzi, V. J., Engert, A., Bradley, E. C., Konrad, M., & Mertelsmann, R. (1988) A phase 1 pilot study of intraperitoneal recombinant interleukin 2 in patients with ovarian carcinoma. *Invest New Drugs* 6:179–188.

Chawla, S. P., Benjamin, R. S., Ayala, A., Carrasco, C. H., Hong, W. K., & Martin, R. G. (1989) Advanced basal cell carcinoma and successful treatment with chemotherapy. *J Surg Oncol* 40:68–72.

Chen, H-S., & Gross, J. F. (1980) Intra-arterial infusion of anticancer drugs: Theoretic aspects of drug delivery and review of responses. *Cancer Treat Rep* 64:31–40.

Chen, K. K., & Rose, C. L. (1952) Nitrite and thiosulfate therapy in cyanide poisoning. *JAMA* 149:113–119.

Cheung, D. K., Regan, J., Savin, M., Gibberman, V., & Woessner, W. (1988) A pilot study of intraarterial chemotherapy with cisplatin in locally advanced head and neck cancers. *Cancer* 61:903–908.

Chu, D. Z. J., Hutchins, L., & Lang, N. P. (1988) Regional chemotherapy of liver metastases from colorectal carcinoma: Hepatic artery or portal vein infusion. *Cancer Treat Rev* 15:243–256.

Chuang, V. P., Benjamin, R., Jaffe, N., Wallace, S., Ayala, A. G., Murray, J., Charnsangavej, C., & Soo, C-S. (1982) Radiographic and angiographic changes in osteosarcoma after intraarterial chemotherapy. *AJR* 139:1065–1069.

Clark, A. W., Cohen, S. R., Nissenblatt, M. J., & Wilson, S. K. (1982) Paraplegia following intrathecal chemotherapy: Neuropathologic findings and elevation of myelin basic protein. *Cancer* 50:42–47.

Clarkson, B. (1964a) Relationship between cell type, glucose concentration, and response to treatment in neoplastic effusions. *Cancer* 17:914–928.

Clarkson, B., O'Connor, A., Winston, L., & Hutchinson, D. (1964b) The physiologic disposition of 5-fluorouracil and 5-fluoro-2'-deoxyuridine in man. *Clin Pharmacol Ther* 5:581–610.

Clarkson, B., Young, C., Dierick, W., Kuehn, P., Kim, M., Berrett, A., Clapp, P., & Lawrence, W., Jr. (1962) Effects of continuous hepatic artery infusion of antimetabolites on primary and metastatic cancer of the liver. *Cancer* 15:472–488.

Cohen, A. M., Kaufman, S. D., & Wood, W. C. (1984) Treatment of colorectal cancer hepatic metastases by hepatic artery chemotherapy. *Dis Colon Rectum* 28:389–393.

Cohen, A. M., Schaeffer, N., & Higgins, J. (1986) Treatment of metastatic colorectal cancer with hepatic artery combination chemotherapy. *Cancer* 57:1115–1117.

Cohen, C. J. (1985) Surgical considerations in ovarian cancer. *Semin Oncol* 12(3; Suppl. 4):53–56.

Coit, D. G., Bajorin, D. F., Menendez-Botet, C., Shiu, M. H., Sclafani, L., Niedzwiecki, D., & Ray, C. (1989) A phase 1 trial of hyperthermic isolation limb perfusion using cisplatin for metastatic intransit melanoma (abstract). *Proc Am Soc Clin Oncol* 8:285.

Colcher, D., Esteban, J., Carrasquillo, J. A., Sugarbaker, P., Reynolds, J. C., Bryant, G., Larson, S. M., & Schlom, J. (1987) Complementation of intracavitary and intravenous administration of a monoclonal antibody (B72.3) in patients with carcinoma. *Cancer Res* 47:4218–4224.

Collins, J. M. (1984) Pharmacokinetic rationale for regional drug delivery. *J Clin Oncol* 2:498–504.

Colombo, N., Speyer, J., Wernz, J., Beckman, E. M., Beller, U., Meyers, M., Canetta, R., & Muggia, F. M. (1987) Phase I–II study of intraperitoneal CBDCA in patients with advanced ovarian cancer (abstract). *Proc Am Soc Clin Oncol* 6:113.

Conway, J. G., Popp, J. A., Ji, S., & Thurman, R. G. (1983) Effect of size on portal circulation of hepatic nodules from carcinogen-treated rats. *Cancer Res* 43:3374–3379.

Conway, J. G., Popp, J. A., & Thurman, R. G. (1985) Microcirculation of hepatic nodules from diethylnitrosamine-treated rats. *Cancer Res* 45:3620–3625.

Copeland, L. J., & Gershenson, D. M. (1986) Ovarian cancer recurrences in patients with no macroscopic tumor at second-look laparotomy. *Obstet Gynecol* 68:873–874.

Copeland, L. J., Gershenson, D. M., Wharton, J. T., Atkinson, E. N., Sneige, N., Edwards, C. L., & Rutledge, F. N. (1985) Microscopic disease at second-look laparotomy in advanced ovarian cancer. *Cancer* 55:472–478.

Creagan, E. T. (1989) Regional and systemic strategies for metastatic malignant melanoma. *Mayo Clin Proc* 64:852–860.

Cumberlin, R., De Moss, E., Lassus, M., & Friedman, M. (1985) Isolation perfusion for malignant melanoma of the extremity: A review. *J Clin Oncol* 3:1022–1031.

D'Acquisto, R., Markman, M., Hakes, T., Rubin, S., Hoskins, W., & Lewis, J. L., Jr. (1988) A phase 1 trial of intraperitoneal recombinant-gamma interferon in advanced ovarian carcinoma. *J Clin Oncol* 6:689–695.

Dakhil, S., Ensminger, W., Cho, K., Niederhuber, J., Doan, K., & Wheeler, R. (1982) Improved regional selectivity of hepatic arterial BCNU with degradable microspheres. *Cancer* 50:631–635.

Daly, J. M., Butler, J., Kemeny, N., Yeh, S. D. J., Ridge, J. A., Botet, J., Bading, J. R., DeCosse, J. J., & Benua, R. S. (1985) Predicting tumor response in patients with colorectal hepatic metastases. *Ann Surg* 202:384–393.

Daly, J. M., Kemeny, N., Oderman, P., & Botet, J. (1984) Long-term hepatic arterial infusion chemotherapy: Anatomic considerations, operative technique, and treatment morbidity. *Arch Surg* 119:936–941.

Daly, J. M., Kemeny, N., Sigurdson, E., Oderman, P., & Thom, A. (1987) Regional infusion for colorectal hepatic metastases: A randomized trial comparing the hepatic artery with the portal vein. *Arch Surg* 112:1273–1277.

Danis, M., Patrick, D. L., Southerland, L. I., & Green, M. L. (1988) Patients' and families' preferences for medical intensive care. *JAMA* 260:797–802.

Daugherty, J. P., LaCreta, F. P., Gibson, N., McGuire, T., Hogan, M., Rosenblum, N., Tew, K., Weese, J. L., & Comis, R. L. (1987) Phase 1 study of intraperitoneal etoposide. *Proc Am Soc Clin Oncol* 6:32.

Dauplat, J., Hacker, N. F., Nieberg, R. K., Berek, J. S., Rose, T. P., & Sagae, S. (1987) Distant metastases in epithelial ovarian carcinoma. *Cancer* 60:1561–1566.

Davis, S., Rambotti, P., & Grignani, F. (1984) Intrapericardial tetracycline sclerosis in the treatment of malignant pericardial effusion: An analysis of thirty-three cases. *J Clin Oncol* 2:631–636.

Dawson, D. M., Rosenthal, D. S., & Maloney, W. C. (1973) Neurological complications of acute leukemia in adults: Changing rate. *Ann Intern Med* 79:541–544.

DeBruyne, F. M. J., van der Meijden A. P. M., Geboers, A. D. H., Franssen M. P. H., van Leeuwen, M. J. W., Steerenberg, P. A., de Jong, W. H., & Ruitenberg, J. J. (1988) BCG (RIVM) versus mitomycin intravesical therapy in superficial bladder cancer: First results of randomized prospective trial. *Urology* 31(Suppl. 3):20–25.

Dedrick, R. L. (1985) Theoretical and experimental bases of intraperitoneal chemotherapy. *Semin Oncol* 12(3; Suppl. 4):1–6.

Dedrick, R. L. (1988) Arterial drug infusion: Pharmacokinetic problems and pitfalls. *JNCI* 80:83–89.

Dedrick, R. L., Myers, C. E., Bungay, P. M., & DeVita, V. T., Jr. (1978) Pharmacokinetic rationale for peritoneal drug administration in the treatment of ovarian cancer. *Cancer Treat Rep* 62:1–9.

DeDycker, R. P., Timmermann, J., Schumacher, T., & Schindler, A. E. (1988) The influence of arterial regional chemotherapy on the local recurrence rate of advanced breast cancer. *Reg Cancer Treat* 1:112–116.

DeGraaf, P. W., Mellema, M. M., Ten Bokkel Huinink, W. W., Aartsen, E. J., Dubbelman, R., Franklin, H. R., & Hart, A. A. (1988) Complications of Tenckhoff catheter implantation in patients with multiple previous intraabdominal procedures for ovarian carcinoma. *Gynecol Oncol* 29(1):43–49.

DeKernion, J. B., Huang, H-Y., Lindner, A., Smith, R. B., & Kaufman, J. J. (1985) The management of superficial bladder tumors and carcinoma in situ with intravesical Bacillus Calmette-Guerin. *J Urol* 133:598–601.

Delgado, G., Potkul, R. K., Treat, J. A., Lewandrowski, G. S., Barter, J. F., Forst, D., & Rahman, A. (1989) A phase I/II study of intraperitoneally administered doxorubicin entrapped in cardiolipin liposomes in patients with ovarian cancer. *Am J Obstet Gynecol* 160:812–819.

Demicheli, R., Bonciarelli, G., Jirillo, A., Foroni, R., Petrosino, L., Targa, L., & Garusi, G. (1985) Pharmacologic data and technical feasibility of intraperitoneal doxorubicin administration. *Tumori* 71:63–68.

Demicheli, R., Jirillo, A., Bonciarelli, G., Bellini, A., Petrosino, L., Bigi, L., & Garusi, G. F. (1982) Pharmacological data and technical feasibility of intraperitoneal 5-fluorouracil administration. *Tumori* 68:437–441.

Deregorio, M. W., Lum, B. L., Holleran, W. M., Wilbur, B. J., & Sikic, B. I. (1986) Preliminary observations of intraperitoneal carboplatin pharmacokinetic during a phase I study of the Northern California Oncology Group. *Cancer Chemother Pharmacol* 18:235–238.

Deutsch, M., Rewers, A. B., Redgate, E. S., Fisher, E. R., & Boggs, S. S. (1989) 5-Iodo-2-deoxyuridine administered into the lateral cerebral ventricle as a radiosensitizer in the treatment of disseminated glioma. *JNCI* 81:1322–1325.

DeWys, W. D., & Fowler, E. H. (1973) Report of vasculitis and blindness after intracarotid infection of 1,3-bis(2-chloroethyl)-1-nitrosurea (BCNU; NSC-409962) in dogs. *Cancer Chemother Rep* 57:33–40.

Dietzel, F. (1983) Basic principles in hyperthermic tumor therapy. *Recent Results Cancer Res* 86:177–190.

DiFilippo, F., Calabro, A., Giannarelli, D., Carlini, S., Cavaliere, F., Moscarelli, F., & Cavaliere, R. (1989) Prognostic variables in recurrent limb melanoma treated with hyperthermic antiblastic perfusion. *Cancer* 63:2551–2561.

Dinndorf, P. A., & Bleyer, W. A. (1987) Management of infectious complications of intraventricular reservoirs in cancer patients: Low incidence and successful treatment without reservoir removal. *Cancer Drug Deliv* 4:105–117.

Doci, R., Bignami, P., Bozzetti, F., Bonfanti, G., Audisio, R., Colombo, M., & Gennari, L. (1988) Intrahepatic chemotherapy for unresectable hepatocellular carcinoma. *Cancer* 61:1983–1987.

Donegan, W. L. (1985) Hepatic artery infusion chemotherapy for colorectal metastases: A personal experience. *J Clin Oncol* 30:177–183.

Donovan, K., Sanson-Fisher, R. W., & Redman, S. (1989) Measuring quality of life in cancer patients. *J Clin Oncol* 7:959–968.

Doria, M. I., Shepard, K. V., Levin, B., & Riddel, R. H. (1986) Liver pathology following hepatic arterial infusion chemotherapy: Hepatic toxicity with FUDR. *Cancer* 58:855–861.

Doroshow, J., Braly, P., Hoff, S., Burgeson, P., Leong, L., Blayney, D., Goldberg, D., Carr, B., Margolin, K., & Akman, S. (1986) Intraperitoneal chemotherapy with cisplatin and 5-fluorouracil: An active regimen for refractory ovarian cancer (abstract). *Proc Am Soc Clin Oncol* 5:117.

Dorr, R. T., Alberts, D. S., & Soble, M. (1986) Lack of experimental vesicant activity for the anticancer agents cisplatin, melphalan, and mitoxantrone. *Cancer Chemother Pharmacol* 16:91–94.

Douglass, H. O. (1985) Gastric cancer: Overview of current therapies. *Semin Oncol* 12(3; Suppl. 4):57–62.

Droller, M. J., & Walsh, P. C. (1985) Intensive intravesical chemotherapy in the treatment of flat carcinoma in situ: Is it safe? *J Urol* 134:1115–1117.

Dunnick, N. R., Jones, R. B., Doppmen, J. L., Speyer, J., & Myers, C. E. (1979) Intraperitoneal contrast infusion for assessment of intraperitoneal fluid dynamics. *AJR* 133:221–223.

Dunton, S. F., Nitschke, R., Spruce, W. E., Bodensteiner, J., & Krous, H. F. (1986) Progressive ascending paralysis following administration of intrathecal and intravenous cytosine arabinoside: A Pediatric Oncology Group study. *Cancer* 57:1083–1088.

Durand, R. E. (1981) Flow cytometry studies of intracellular adriamycin in multicell spheroids in vitro. *Cancer Res* 41:3495–3498.

Duttera, M. J., Bleyer, W. A., Pomeroy, T. C., Leventhal, C. M., & Leventhal, B. G. (1973) Irradiation, methotrexate toxicity, and the treatment of meningeal leukemia. *Lancet* 2:703–707.

Eapen, L., Stewart, D., Danjoux, C., Genest, P., Futter, N., Moors, D., Irvine, A., Crook, J., Aitken, S., Gerig, L., Peterson, R., & Rasuli, P. (1989) Intraarterial cisplatin and concurrent radiation for locally advanced bladder cancer. *J Clin Oncol* 7:230–235.

Edmonson, J. H., Decker, D. G., Malkasian, G. D., Webb, M. J., & Jorgensen, E. O. (1978) Phase II evaluation of VP-16-213 (NSC-141540) in patients with advanced ovarian carcinoma resistant to alkylating agents. *Gynecol Oncol* 6:7–9.

Eggermont, A. M. M. (1989) Intracavitary immunotherapy: Past, present, and future treatment strategies. *Reg Cancer Treat* 2:37–48.

Eilber, F. R., Grant, T., & Morton, D. L. (1978) Adjuvant therapy for osteosarcoma: Preoperative and postoperative treatment. *Cancer Treat Rep* 62:213–216.

Eilber, F. R., Mirra, J. J., Grant, T. T., Weisenburger, T., & Morton, D. L. (1980) Is amputation necessary for sarcomas? A seven-year experience with limb salvage. *Ann Surg* 192:431–438.

Eilber, F. R., Morton, D. L., Eckardt, J., Grant, T., & Weisenburger, T. (1984) Limb salvage for skeletal and soft tissue sarcomas: Multidisciplinary preoperative therapy. *Cancer* 53:2579–2584.

Einhorn, L. H., & Donohue, J. (1977) Cis-diamminedichloroplatinum, vinblastine, and bleomycin combination chemotherapy in disseminated testicular cancer. *Ann Intern Med* 87:293–298.

Ekberg, H., Tranberg, K. G., Persson, B., Jeppsson, B., Nilsson, L. G., Gustafson, T., Andersson, K. E., & Bengmark, S. (1988) Intraperitoneal infusion of 5-FU in liver metastases from colorectal cancer. *J Surg Oncol* 37:94–99.

Elferink, F., van der Vijgh, W. J., Klein, I., Ten Bokkel Huinink, W. W., Dubbelman, R., & McVie, J. G. (1988) Pharmacokinetics of carboplatin after intraperitoneal administration. *Cancer Chemother Pharmacol* 21(1):57–60.

Elmes, P. C., & Simpson, M. J. C. (1976) The clinical aspects of mesothelioma. *Q J Med* 45:427–449.

Ensminger, W. (1989) Hepatic arterial chemotherapy for primary and metastatic liver cancers. *Cancer Chemother Pharmacol* 23(Suppl.):S68–S73.

Ensminger, W. D., & Gyves, J. W. (1983) Clinical pharmacology of hepatic arterial chemotherapy. *Semin Oncol* 10:176–182.

Ensminger, W. D., Gyves, J. W., Stetson, P., & Walker-Andrews, S. (1985) Phase 1 study of hepatic arterial degradable starch microspheres and mitomycin. *Cancer Res* 45:4464–4467.

Ensminger, W., Niederhuber, J., Dakhil, S., Thrall, J., & Wheeler, R. (1981) Totally implanted drug delivery system for hepatic arterial chemotherapy. *Cancer Treat Rep* 65:393–400.

Ensminger, W. D., Rosowsky, A., Raso, V., Levin, D. C., Glode, M., Come, S., Steele, G., & Frei, E. (1978) A clinical-pharmacological evaluation of hepatic arterial infusions of 5-fluoro-2'-deoxyuridine and 5-fluorouracil. *Cancer Res* 38:3784–3792.

Epenetos, A. A. (1984) Antibody-guided irradiation of malignant lesions: Three cases illustrating a new method of treatment. *Lancet* 1:1441–1443.

Epenetos, A. A. (1985) Clinical results with regional antibody-guided irradiation. *Cancer Drug Deliv* 2:233.

Epenetos, A. A., Munro, A. J., Stewart, S., Rampling, R., Lambert, H. E., McKenzie, C. G., Soutter, P., Rahemtulla, A., Hooker, G., Sivolapenko, G. B., Snook, D., Courtenay-Luck, N., Dhokia, B., Krausz, T., Taylor-Papadimitriou, J., & Bodmer, W. F. (1987) Antibody-guided irradiation of advanced ovarian cancer with intraperitoneally administered radiolabeled monoclonal antibodies. *J Clin Oncol* 5:1890–1899.

Esposito, M., Campora, E., Repetto, M., Fulco, R. A., Simoni, G. A., Falcone, A., Collecchi, P., Gogioso, L., Nobile, M. T., & Civalleri, D. (1988) Regional pharmacokinetic selectivity of intraperitoneal cisplatin in ovarian cancer. *Oncology* 45(2):69–73.

Fanning, J., Daugherty, J. P., & Weese, J. L. (1989) Resolution of malignant small bowel obstruction after intraperitoneal etoposide therapy. *South Med J* 82:798–799.

Fentiman, I. S. (1987) Diagnosis and treatment of malignant pleural effusions. *Cancer Treat Rev* 14:107–118.

Fer, M. F., Weiden, P. L., Morgan, A. C., Sivam, G., Yon, J., Schroff, R. W., Appelbaum, J. A., Bjorn, M., Manger, R., & Abrams, P. G. (1989) Pseudomonas exotoxin A-monoclonal antibody conjugates: A phase 1 study in peritoneal metastases (abstract). *Proc Am Soc Clin Oncol* 8:165.

Ferraris, V. (1988) Doxorubicin plus mitomycin C regimen in the prophylactic treatment of superficial bladder tumors. *Cancer* 62:1055–1060.

Feun, L. G., Lee, Y-Y., Yung, A., Charnsangavej, C., Savaraj, N., Tang, R. A., & Wallace, S. (1986) Phase II trial of intracarotid BCNU and cisplatin in primary malignant brain tumors. *Cancer Drug Deliv* 3:147–155.

Feun, L. G., Wallace, S., Stewart, D. J., Chuang, V. P., Yung, W-K. A., Levens, M. E., Burgess, M. A., Savaraj, N., Benjamin, R. S., Young, S. E., Tang, R. A., Handel, S., Mavligit, G., & Fields, W. S. (1984) Intracarotid infusion of cis-diamminedichloroplatinum in the treatment of recurrent malignant brain tumors. *Cancer* 54:794–799.

Feun, L. G., Wallace, S., Yung, W-K. A., Lee, Y. Y., Leavens, M. E., Moser, R., Savaraj, N., Burgess, M. A., Plager, C., Benjamin, R. S., Tang, R. A., Mavligit, G. M., & Fields, W. S. (1984) Phase I trial of intracarotid BCNU and cisplatin in patients with malignant intracerebral tumors. *Cancer Drug Deliv* 1:239–245.

Finkler, N. J., Muto, M. G., Kassis, A. I., Weadock, K., Tumeh, S. S., Zurawski, V. R., & Knapp, R. C. (1989) Intraperitoneal radiolabeled OC 125 in patients with advanced ovarian cancer. *Gynecol Oncol* 34:339–344.

Fiorentino, M. V., Daniele, O., Morandi, P., Aversa, S. M. L., Ghiotto, C., Paccagnella, A., & Fornasiero, A. (1988) Intrapericardial instillation of platin in malignant pericardial effusion. *Cancer* 62:1904–1905.

Fisher, R. I., DeVita, V. T., Hubbard, S. P., Simon, R., & Young, R. C. (1979) Prolonged disease-free survival in Hodgkin's disease with MOPP reinduction after first relapse. *Ann Intern Med* 90:761–763.

Fleischmann, J. D., Toossi, Z., Ellner, J. J., Wentworth, D. B., Ratliff, T. L., & Imbembo, A. L. (1989) Urinary interleukins in patients receiving intravesical Bacillus Calmette-Guerin therapy for superficial bladder cancer. *Cancer* 64:1447–1454.

Flowerdew, A. D. S., McLaren, M. I., Fleming, J. S., Britten, A. J., Ackery, D. M., Birch, S. J., Taylor, I., & Karran, S. J. (1987) Liver tumour blood flow and responses to arterial embolization measured by dynamic hepatic scintigraphy. *Br J Cancer* 55:269–273.

Forastiere, A. A., Baker, S. R., Wheeler, R., & Medvek, B. R. (1987) Intra-arterial cisplatin and FUDR in advanced malignancies confined to the head and neck. *J Clin Oncol* 5:1601–1606.

Fortner, J. G., Silva, J. S., Golbey, R. B., Cox, E. B., & Maclean, B. J. (1984) Multivariate analysis of a personal series of 247 consecutive patients with liver metastases from colorectal cancer. *Ann Surg* 199:303–316.

Franklin, H. R., Koops, H. S., Oldhoff, J., Czarnetzki, B. M., Macher, E., Kroon, B. B. R., Welvaart, K., van der Velden, J. W., van Dijk, E., van der Esch, E. P., Oosterhuis, J. W., Huisman, S. J., Hart, A. A. M., & Rumke, P. (1988) To perfuse or not to perfuse? A retrospective study to evaluate the effect of adjuvant isolated regional perfusion in patients with stage I extremity melanoma with a thickness of 1.5 mm or greater. *J Clin Oncol* 6:701–708.

Freckman, H. A. (1972) Results in 169 patients with cancer of the head and neck treated by intra-arterial infusion therapy. *Am J Surg* 124:501–509.

Frei, E., & Canellos, G. P. (1980) Dose: A critical factor in cancer chemotherapy. *Am J Med* 69:585–594.

Frustaci, S., Barzan, L., Tumolo, S., Comoretto, R., Quadu, G., Galligioni, E., Lorenzini, M., Crivellari, D., Caruso, G., Piccinin, G., Veronesi, A., Tirelli, U., & Grigoletto, E. (1986) Intra-arterial continuous infusion of cis-diamminedichloroplatinum in untreated head and neck cancer patients. *Cancer* 57:1118–1123.

Fujimoto, S., Shrestha, R. D., Kokubun, M., Kobayashi, D., Kiuchi, S., Takahashi, M., Konno, C., Ohta, M., Koike, S., Kitsukawa, Y., Mizutani, M., & Okui, K. (1989) Clinical trial with surgery and intraperitoneal hyperthermic perfusion for peritoneal recurrence of gastrointestinal cancer. *Cancer* 64:154–160.

Fujimoto, S., Shrestha, R. D., Kokubun, M., Kobayashi, D., Kiuchi, S., Takahashi, M., Konno, C., Ohta, M., Koike, S., Kitsukawa, Y., Mizutani, M., & Okui, K. (1989) itoneal hyperthermic perfusion combined with surgery effective for gastric cancer patients with peritoneal seeding. *Ann Surg* 208:36–41.

Fujiwara, K, Tamada, T., Mizutani, Y., Hayase, R., Kohno, I., & Sekiba, K. (1989) Intraperitoneal mitomycin C as first-line treatment of ovarian carcinoma correlated with human tumor clonogenic assay findings (abstract). *Proc Am Soc Clin Oncol* 8:156.

Fuller, D. B., Sause, W. T., Plenk, H. P., & Menlove, R. L. (1987) Analysis of postoperative radiation therapy in Stage I through III epithelial ovarian carcinoma. *J Clin Oncol* 5:897–905.

Ganz, P. A., Haskell, C. M., Figlin, R. A., LaSoto, N., & Sias, J. (1988) Estimating the quality of life in a clinical trial of patients with metastatic lung cancer using the Karnofsky Performance Status and the Functional Living Index—Cancer. *Cancer* 61:849–856.

Garnick, M. B., Schade, D., Israel, M., Maxwell, B., & Richie, J. P. (1984) Intravesical doxorubicin for prophylaxis in the management of superficial bladder carcinoma. *J Urol* 131:43–46.

Geisler, H. E. (1983) Megestrol acetate for the palliation of advanced ovarian carcinoma. *Obstet Gynecol* 61:95–98.

Ghussen, F., Kruger, I., Groth, W., & Stutzer, H. (1988) The role of regional hyperthermic cytostatic perfusion in the treatment of extremity melanoma. *Cancer* 61:654–659.

Ghussen, F., Nagel, K., Groth, W., Muller, J. M., & Stutzer, H. (1984) A prospective randomized study of regional extremity perfusion in patients with malignant melanoma. *Ann Surg* 200:764–768.

Ghussen, F., Nagel, K., & Isselhard, W. (1983) Isolated liver perfusion in dogs. *Recent Results Cancer Res* 86:93–98.

Gianni, L., Jenkins, J. F., Greene, R. F., Lichter, A. S., Myers, C. E., & Collins, J. M. (1983) Pharmacokinetics of the hypoxic radiosensitizers misonidazole and demethylmisonidazole after intraperitoneal administration in humans. *Cancer Res* 43:913–916.

Giannone, L., Greco, F. A., & Hainsworth, J. D. (1986) Combination intraventricular chemotherapy for meningeal neoplasia. *J Clin Oncol* 4:68–73.

Gianola, F. J., Sugarbaker, P. H., Barofsky, I., White, D. E., & Myers, C. E. (1986) Toxicity studies of adjuvant intravenous versus intraperitoneal 5-FU in patients with advanced primary colon or rectal cancer. *Am J Clin Oncol* 9:403–410.

Giovanellia, B. C., Stehlin, J. S., Jr., & Morgan, A. C. (1976) Selective lethal effect of supranormal temperatures on human neoplastic cells. *Cancer Res* 36:3944–3950.

Goel, R., Cleary, S. M., Horton, C., Balis, F. M., Zimm, S., Kirmani, S., & Howell, S. B. (1989) Selective intraperitoneal biochemical modulation of methotrexate by dipyridamole. *J Clin Oncol* 7:262–269.

Goldie, J. H., & Coldman, A. J. (1979) A mathematical model for relating the drug sensitivity of tumors to their spontaneous mutation rate. *Cancer Treat Rep* 63:1727–1733.

Goldie, J. H., Coldman, A. J., & Gudauskas, G. A. (1982) Rationale for the use of alternating non-cross-resistant chemotherapy. *Cancer Treat Rep* 66:439–449.

Goldman, M. L., Bilbao, M. K., Rosch, J., & Dotter, C. T. (1975) Complications of indwelling chemotherapy catheters. *Cancer* 36:1983–1990.

Goodwin, P. J., Feld, R., Evans, W. K., & Pater, J. (1988) Cost-effectiveness of cancer chemotherapy: An economic evaluation of a randomized trial in small-cell lung cancer. *J Clin Oncol* 6:1537–1547.

Gouyette, A., Apchin, A., Foka, M., & Richards, J-M. (1986) Pharmacokinetics of intra-arterial and intravenous cisplatin in head and neck cancer patients. *Eur J Cancer Clin Oncol* 22:257–263.

Grage, T. B., Vassilopoulos, P. P., Shingelton, W. W., Jubert, A. V., Elias, E. G., Aust, J. B., & Moss, S. E. (1979) Results of a prospective randomized study of hepatic artery infusion with 5-fluorouracil versus intravenous 5-fluorouracil in patients with hepatic metastases from colorectal cancer: A Central Oncology Group study. *Surgery* 86:550–555.

Green, D. M., West, C. R., Brecher, M. L., Ettinger, L. J., Bakshi, S., Berger, P., Parthasarathy, K. L., & Freeman, A. I. (1982) The use of subcutaneous cerebrospinal fluid reservoirs for the prevention and treatment of meningeal relapse of acute lymphoblastic leukemia. *Am J Pediatr Hematol Oncol* 4:147–154.

Green, T. H. (1959) Hemisulfur mustard in the palliation of patients with metastatic ovarian carcinoma. *Obstet Gynecol* 13:383–393.

Greenberg, H. S., Ensminger, W. D., Seeger, J. F., Kindt, G. W., Chandler, W. F., Doan, K., & Dakhil, S. R. (1981) Intra-arterial BCNU chemotherapy for the treatment of malignant gliomas of the central nervous system: A preliminary report. *Cancer Treat Rep* 65:803–810.

Grem, J. L., Hoth, D. F., Hamilton, J. M., King, S. A., & Leyland-Jones, B. (1987) Overview of current status and future direction of clinical trials with 5-fluorouracil in combination with folinic acid. *Cancer Treat Rep* 71:1249–1264.

Griffin, J. W., Thompson, R. W., Mitchinson, M. J., de Kiewiet, J. C., & Welland, F. H. (1971) Lymphomatous leptomeningitis. *Am J Med* 51:200–208.

Grossman, S. A., Trump, D. L., Chen, D. C. P., Thompson, G., & Camargo, E. E. (1982) Cerebrospinal fluid flow abnormalities in patients with neoplastic meningitis: An evaluation using ^{111}indium-DTPA ventriculography. *Am J Med* 73:641–647.

Guinan, P., Brosman, S., DeKernion, J., Lamm, D., Williams, R., Richardson, C., Reitsma, D., & Hanna, M. (1989) Intravesical Bacillus Calmette-Guerin and second primary malignancies. *Urology* 33:380–381.

Guinan, P., Crispen, R., & Rubenstein, M. (1987) BCG in management of superficial bladder cancer. *Urology* 30:515–519.

Guinan, P., Shaw, M., & Ray, V. (1986) Histopathology of BCG and thiotepa treated bladders. *Urol Res* 14:211–215.

Gupta, R. C., Lavengood, R., & Smith, J. P. (1988) Miliary tuberculosis due to intravesical Bacillus Calmette-Guerin therapy. *Chest* 94:1296–1298.

Gutin, P. H., Green, M. R., Bleyer, W. A., Bauer, V. L., Wiernik, P. H., & Walker, M. D. (1976) Methotrexate pneumonitis induced by intrathecal methotrexate therapy: A case report with pharmacokinetic data. *Cancer* 38:1529–1534.

Gutin, P. H., Levi, J. A., Wiernik, P. H., & Walker, M. D. (1977) Treatment of malignant meningeal disease with intrathecal thiotepa: A phase II study. *Cancer Treat Rep* 61:885–887.

Gutin, P. H., Weiss, H. D., Wiernik, P. H., & Walker, M. D. (1976) Intrathecal N,N',N' triethylenethiophosphoramide (thio-tepa (NSC 6396)) in the treatment of malignant meningeal disease: Phase I–II study. *Cancer* 38:1471–1475.

Gyves, J. (1985) Pharmacology of intraperitoneal infusion 5-fluorouracil and mitomycin-c *Semin Oncol* 12(3; Suppl. 4):29–32.

Gyves, J. W., Ensminger, W. D., Stetson, P., Niederhuber, J. E., Meyer, M., Walker, S., Janis, M. A., & Gilbertson, S., (1984) Constant intraperitoneal 5-fluorouracil infusion through a totally implanted system. *Clin Pharmacol Ther* 35:83–89.

Haaff, E. O., Catalona, W. J., & Batliff, T. L. (1986) Detection of interleukin 2 in the urine of patients with superficial bladder tumors after treatment with intravesical BCG. *J Urol* 136:970–974.

Haaxma-Reiche, H., & Van Imhoff, G. W. (1989) Results of intraventricular central nervous system prophylaxis and treatment in non-Hodgkin's lymphoma. *Reg Cancer Treat* 2:32–36.

Hacker, N. F., Berek, J. S., Pretorius, R. G., Zuckerman, J., Eisenkop, S., & Lagasse, L. D. (1987) Intraperitoneal cis-platinum as salvage therapy for refractory epithelial ovarian cancer. *Obstet Gynecol* 70:759–764.

Hafstrom, L., Jonsson, P-E., Landberg, T., Owman, T., & Sundkvist, K. (1979) Intraarterial infusion chemotherapy (5-fluorouracil) in patients with inextirpable or locally recurrent rectal cancer. *Am J Surg* 137:757–762.

Haghbin, M., & Galicich, J. H. (1979) Use of the Ommaya reservoir in the prevention and treatment of CNS leukemia. *Am J Pediatr Hematol Oncol* 1:111–117.

Hagiwara, A., Takahashi, T., Ueda, T., Lee, R., Takeda, M., & Itoh, T., (1988) Intraoperative chemotherapy with carbon particles absorbing mitomycin C for gastric cancer with peritoneal dissemination in rabbits. *Surgery* 104:874–881.

Hahn, G. M. (1979) Potential for therapy of drugs and hyperthermia. *Cancer Res* 39:2264–2268.

Haisma, H. J., Moseley, K. R., Battaile, A., Griffiths, T. C., & Knapp, R. C. (1988) Distribution and pharmacokinetics of radiolabeled monoclonal antibody OC 125 after intravenous and intraperitoneal administration in gynecology tumors. *Am J Obstet Gynecol* 159:843–848.

Hakes, T. B., Chalas, E., Saigo, P., Geller, N., & Lewis, J. L. (1987) Randomized prospective trial of cyclophosphamide, doxorubicin, and cisplatin chemotherapy: 5 versus 10 cycles in stage III & IV ovarian carcinoma (abstract). *Proc Am Soc Clin Oncol* 6:116.

Hakes, T., Markman, M., Reichman, T., Hoskins, W., Jones, W., Rubin, S., Almadrones, L., & Lewis, J. L. (1989) High intensity intravenous cyclophosphamide/cisplatin & intraperitoneal cisplatin for advanced ovarian cancer (abstract). *Proc Am Soc Clin Oncol* 8:152.

Hanks, J. B., & Jones, R. S. (1986) The pathogenesis, detection, and surgical treatment of hepatic metastases. *Curr Probl Cancer* 10:216–265.

Harari, P. M., Shimm, D. S., Gerner, E. W., & Alberts, D. S. (1989) Intraperitoneal chemotherapy plus regional/systemic hyperthermia in the treatment of advanced ovarian cancer. *Reg Cancer Treat* 2:54–58.

Hardeman, S. W., Perry, A., & Soloway, M. S. (1988) Transitional cell carcinoma of the prostate following intravesical therapy for transitional cell carcinoma of the bladder. *J Urol* 140:289–292.

Hausheer, F. H., & Yarbro, J. W. (1985) Diagnosis and treatment of malignant pleural effusion. *Semin Oncol* 12:54–75.

Head and Neck Contracts Program. (1987) Adjuvant chemotherapy for advanced head and neck squamous carcinoma: Final report of the Head and Neck Contracts Program. *Cancer* 60:301–311.

Heim, M. E., Eberwein, S., & Georgi, M. (1983) Palliative therapy of pelvic tumors by intra-arterial infusion of cytotoxic drugs. *Recent Results Cancer Res* 86:38–40.

Heintz, A. P. M., Hacker, N. F., Berek, J. S., Rose, T. P., Munoz, A. K., & Lagasse, L. D. (1986) Cytoreductive surgery in ovarian carcinoma: Feasibility and morbidity. *Obstet Gynecol* 67:783–788.

Heney, N. M. (1988) Intravesical chemotherapy: How effective is it? *Urology* 31(Suppl. 3):17–19.

Heney, N. M., Koontz, W. W., Barton, B., Soloway, M., Trump, D. L., Hazra, T., & Weinstein, R. S. (1988) Intravesical thiotepa versus mitomycin C in patients with TA, T1 and TIS transitional cell carcinoma of the bladder: A phase III prospective randomized study. *J Urol* 140:1390–1393.

Herba, M. J., Illescas, F. F., Thirlwell, M. P., Boos, G. J., Rosenthall, L., Atri, M., & Bret, P. M. (1988) Hepatic malignancies: Improved treatment with intraarterial Y-90. *Radiology* 169:311–314.

Herr, H. W., Laudone, V. P., Badalment, R. A., Oettgen, H. F., Sogani, P. C., Freedman, B. D., Melamed, M. R., & Whitmore, W. F., Jr. (1988) Bacillus Calmette-Guerin therapy alters the progression of superficial bladder cancer. *J Clin Oncol* 6:1450–1455.

Herr, H. W., Pinsky, C. M., Whitmore, W. F., Jr., Sogani, P. C., Oettgen, H. F., & Melamed, M. R. (1985) Experience with intravesical Bacillus Calmette-Guerin therapy of superficial bladder tumors. *Urology* 25:119–123.

Herr, H. W., Pinsky, C. M., Whitmore, W. F., Jr., Sogani, P. C., Oettgen, H. F., & Melamed, M. R. (1986) Long-term effect of intravesical Bacillus Calmette-Guerin on flat carcinoma in situ of the bladder. *J Urol* 135:265–267.

Hidalgo, V., Hidalgo, O. F., & Calvo, F. A. (1987) Simultaneous radiotherapy and cisplatinum for the treatment of brain metastases: A pilot study. *Am J Clin Oncol* 10:205–209.

Hitchins, R. N., Bell, D. R., Woods, R. L., & Levi, J. A. (1987) A prospective randomized trial of single-agent versus combination chemotherapy in meningeal carcinomatosis. *J Clin Oncol* 5:1655–1662.

Hodgson, W. J. B., Friedland, M., Ahmed, T., Mittelman, A., Berman, H., Katz, S., Morgan, J., & Byrne, D. (1986) Treatment of colorectal hepatic metastases by intrahepatic chemotherapy alone or as an adjuvant to complete or partial removal of metastatic disease. *Ann Surg* 203:420–425.

Hoekstra, H. J., Koops, H. S., Molenaar, W. M., Mehta, D. M., Sleijfer, D. T., Dijkhuis, G., & Oldhoff, J. (1989) A combination of intraarterial chemotherapy, preoperative and postoperative radiotherapy, and surgery as limb-saving treatment of primarily unresectable high-grade soft tissue sarcomas of the extremities. *Cancer* 63:59–62.

Hoekstra, H. J., Koops, H. S., Molenaar, W. M., & Oldhoff, J. (1987) Results of isolated regional perfusion in the treatment of malignant soft tissue tumors of the extremities. *Cancer* 60:1703–1707.

Hohn, D., Melnick, J., Stagg, R., Altman, D., Friedman, M., Ignoffo, R., Ferrell, L., & Lewis, B. (1985) Biliary sclerosis in patients receiving hepatic arterial infusions of floxuridine. *J Clin Oncol* 3:98–102.

Hohn, D. S., Rayner, A. A., Economou, J. S., Ignoffo, R. J., Lewis, B. J., & Stagg, R. J. (1986) Toxicities and complications of implanted pump hepatic arterial and intravenous floxuridine infusion. *Cancer* 57:465–470.

Hohn, D. S., Stagg, R. J., Friedman, M., Hannigan, J. F., Rayner, A., Ignoffo, R. J., Acord, P., & Lewis, B. J. (1989) A randomized trial of continuous intravenous versus hepatic intraarterial floxuridine in patients with colorectal cancer metastatic to the liver: The Northern California Oncology Group trial. *J Clin Oncol* 7:1646–1654.

Hohn, D. S., Stagg, R. J., Price, D. C., & Lewis, B. J. (1985) Avoidance of gastroduodenal toxicity in patients receiving hepatic arterial 5-fluoro-2'-deoxyuridine. *J Clin Oncol* 3:1257–1260.

Holcenberg, J., Anderson, T., Ritch, P., Skibba, J., Howser, D., Ring, B., Adams, S., & Helmsworth, M. (1983) Intraperitoneal chemotherapy with melphalan plus glutaminase. *Cancer Res* 43:1381–1388.

Hollister, D., Jr., & Coleman, M. (1980) Hematologic effects of intravesicular thiotepa therapy for bladder carcinoma. *JAMA* 244:2065–2067.

Hong, F., & Mayhew, E. (1989) Therapy of central nervous system leukemia in mice by liposome-entrapped 1-B-D-arabinofuranosylcytosine. *Cancer Res* 45:5097–5102.

Hong, W. K., & Bromer, R. (1983) Chemotherapy in head and neck cancer. *N Engl J Med* 308:75–79.

Hoskins, W. J., Lichter, A. S., Whittington, R., Artman, L. E., Bibro, M. C., & Park, R. C. (1985) Whole abdominal and pelvic irradiation in patients with minimal disease of second-look surgical assessment for ovarian carcinoma. *Gynecol Oncol* 20:271–280.

Hoskins, W. J., Rubin, S. C., Dulaney, E., Chapman, D., Almadrones, L., Saigo, P., Markman, M., Hakes, T., Reichman, B., Jones, W. B., & Lewis, J. L., Jr. (1989) Influence of secondary cytoreduction at the time of second-look laparotomy on the survival of patients with epithelial ovarian carcinoma. *Gynecol Oncol* 34:365–371.

Howell, S. B., Chu, B. C. F., Wung, W. E., Metha, B. M., & Mendelsohn, J. (1981) Long-duration intracavitary infusion of methotrexate with systemic leucovorin protection in patients with malignant effusion. *J Clin Invest* 67:1161–1170.

Howell, S. B., Kirmani, S., Lucas, W. E., Zimm, S., Goel, R., Kim, S., Horton, M. C., McVey, L., Morris, J., & Weiss, R. J. (1990) A phase II trial of intraperitoneal cisplatin and etoposide for primary treatment of ovarian epithelial cancer. *J Clin Oncol* 8:137–145.

Howell, S. B., Pfeifle, C. E., & Olshen, R. A. (1984) Intraperitoneal chemotherapy with melphalan. *Ann Intern Med* 101:14–18.

Howell, S. B., Pfeifle, C. E., Wung, W. E., & Olshen, R. A. (1983) Intraperitoneal cisplatin with systemic thiosulfate protection. *Cancer Res* 43:1426–1431.

Howell, S. B., Pfeifle, C. E., Wung, W. E., Olshen, R. A., Lucas, W. E., Yon, J. L., & Green, M. (1982) Intraperitoneal cisplatin with systemic thiosulfate protection. *Ann Intern Med* 97:845–851.

Howell, S. B., Schiefer, M., Andrews, P. A., Markman, M., & Abramson, I. (1987) The pharmacology of intraperitoneally administered bleomycin. *J Clin Oncol* 5: 2009–2016.

Howell, S. B., & Taetle, R. (1980) Effect of sodium thiosulfate on cis-diamminedichloroplatinum(II) toxicity and antitumor activity in L1210 leukemia. *Cancer Treat Rep* 64:611–616.

Howell, S. B., Zimm, S., Markman, M., Abramson, I. S., Cleary, S., Lucas, W. E., & Weiss, R. J. (1987) Long term survival of advanced refractory ovarian carcinoma patients with small-volume disease treated with intraperitoneal chemotherapy. *J Clin Oncol* 5:1607–1612.

Hu, E., & Howell, S. B. (1983) Pharmacokinetics of intraarterial mitomycin C in humans. *Cancer Res* 43:4474–4477.

Huberman, M. S. (1983) Comparison of systemic chemotherapy with hepatic arterial infusion in metastatic colorectal carcinoma. *Semin Oncol* 10:238–248.

Huland, E. & Huland, H. (1989) Local continuous high dose interleukin 2: A new therapeutic model for the treatment of advanced bladder carcinoma. *Cancer Res* 49:5469–5474.

Huland, H., Otto, U., Droese, M., & Kloppel, G. (1984) Long-term mitomycin C instillation after transurethral resection of superficial bladder carcinoma: Influence on recurrence, progression and survival. *J Urol* 132:27–29.

Ichihara, T., Sakamoto, K., Mori, K., & Akagi, M. (1989) Transcatheter arterial chemoembolization therapy for hepatocellular carcinoma using polyactic acid microspheres containing aclarubicin hydrochloride. *Cancer Res* 49:4357–4362.

Iitsuka, Y., Kaneshima, S., Tanida, O., Takeuchi, T., & Koga, S. (1979) Intraperitoneal free cancer cells and their viability in gastric cancer. *Cancer* 44:1476–1480.

Issell, B. F., Prout, G. R., Jr., Soloway, M. S., Cummings, K. B., Brannen, G., Veenema, R., Flanagan, M., Block, N. L., Summers, J. L., Levin, E. A., & Defuria, M. D. (1984) Mitomycin C intravesical therapy in noninvasive bladder cancer after failure of thiotepa. *Cancer* 53:1025–1028.

Jacobi, G. H., & Kurth, K-H. (1980) Studies on the intravesical action of topically administered G³H-doxorubicin hydrochloride in men: Plasma uptake and tumor penetration. *J Urol* 124:34–37.

Jacobs, S. C., McCellan, S. L., Maher, C., & Lawson, R. K. (1984) Pre-cystectomy intra-arterial cis-diamminedichloroplatinum II with local bladder hyperthermia for bladder cancer. *J Urol* 131:473–476.

Jacobs, S. C., Menasche, D. S., Mewissen, M. W., & Lipchik, E. O. (1989) Intraarterial cisplatin infusion in the management of transitional cell carcinoma of the bladder. *Cancer* 64:388–391.

Jaffe, N., Knapp, J., Chuang, V. P., Wallace, S., Ayala, A., Murray, J., Cangir, A., Wang, A., & Benjamin, R. S. (1983) Osteosarcoma: Intra-arterial treatment of the primary tumor with cis-diammine-dichloroplatinum II (CDP). *Cancer* 51:402–407.

Jaffe, N., Prudich, J., Knapp, J., Wang, Y-M., Bowman, R., Cangir, A., Ayala, A., Chuang, V., & Wallace, S. (1983) Treatment of primary osteosarcoma with intra-arterial and intravenous high-dose methotrexate. *J Clin Oncol* 1:428–431.

Jaffe, N., Raymond, A. K., Ayala, A., Carrasco, C. H., Wallace, S., Robertson, R., Griffiths, M., & Wang, Y-M. (1989) Effect of cumulative courses of intraarterial cis-diamminedichloroplatinum-II on the primary tumor in osteosarcoma. *Cancer* 63:63–67.

Jaffe, N., Robertson, R., Ayala, A., Wallace, S., Chuang, V., Anzai, T., Cangir, A., Wang, Y-M., & Chen, T. (1985) Comparison of intra-arterial cis-diamminedichloroplatinum II with high-dose methotrexate and citrovorum factor rescue in the treatment of primary osteosarcoma. *J Clin Oncol* 3:1101–1104.

Jaffe, N., Watts, H., Fellows, K. E., & Vawter, G. (1978) Local en bloc resection for limb preservation. *Cancer Treat Rep* 62:217–223.

Janis, L. W., Leming, P. D., & Leder, W. (1988) Nonspecific corticosteroid therapy in patients receiving intra-arterial chemotherapy for hepatic metastases of colorectal origin. *Cancer Invest* 6:267–270.

Janoff, K. A., Moseson, D., Nohlgren, J., Davenport, C., Richards, C., & Fletcher, W. S. (1982) The treatment of stage 1 melanoma of the extremities with regional hyperthermic isolation perfusion. *Ann Surg* 196:316–323.

Jansen, R. F. M., Van Geel, B. N., Van Der Zee, J., Hagenbeek, A., & Levendag, P. C. (1989) Intractable cutaneous non-Hodgkin's lymphoma of the lower limb: Complete remission after sequential regional isolated hyperthermic perfusion and perfusion with 1-phenylalanine-mustard (mephalan, L-PAM). *Cancer* 64:392–395.

Jenkins, J., Sugarbaker, P. H., Gianola, F. J., & Myers, C. E. (1982) Technical considerations in the use of intraperitoneal chemotherapy administered by Tenckhoff catheter. *Surg Gynecol Obstet* 154:858–864.

Jones, H. C., & Swinney, J. (1961) Thio-TEPA in the treatment of tumours of the bladder. *Lancet* 2:615–618.

Jones, R. B., Collins, J. M., Myers, C. E., Brooks, A. E., Hubbard, S., Balow, J. E., Brennan, M. R., Dedrick, R. L., & DeVita, V. T. (1981) High-volume intraperitoneal chemotherapy with methotrexate in patients with cancer. *Cancer Res* 41:55–59.

Julian, C. G., Inalsingh, C. H. A., & Burnett, L. S. (1978) Radioactive phosphorus and external radiation as an adjuvant to surgery for ovarian carcinoma. *Obstet Gynecol* 52:155–160.

Kahn, C., Messersmith, R. N., & Samuels, B. L. (1989) Brachial plexopathy as a complication of intraarterial cisplatin chemotherapy. *Cardiovasc Intervent Radiol* 12:47–49.

Kamada, M., Sakamoto, Y., Furumoto, H., Mori, K., Daitoh, T., Irahara, M., Aono, T., Nii, A., Yanagawa, H., Sonee, S., & Ogura, T. (1989) Treatment of malignant ascites with allogeneic and autologous lymphokine-activated killer cells. *Gynecol Oncol* 34:34–37.

Kane, M. J. (1989) Chemotherapy of advanced soft tissue and osteosarcomas. *Semin Oncol* 16:297–304.

Kaplan, R. A., Markman, M., Lucas, W. E., Pfeifle, C., & Howell, S. B. (1985) Infectious peritonitis in patients receiving intraperitoneal chemotherapy. *Am J Med* 78:49–53.

Kaplan, W. D., Ensminger, W. D., Come, S. E., Smith, E. H., D'Orsi, C. J., Levin, D. C., Takvorian, R. W., & Steele, G. D., Jr. (1980) Radionuclide angiography to predict patient response to hepatic artery chemotherapy. *Cancer Treat Res* 64: 1217–1222.

Kar, R., Cohen, R. A., Terem, T. M., Nahabedian, M. Y., & Wile, A. G. (1986) Pharmacokinetics of 5-fluorouracil in rabbits in experimental regional chemotherapy. *Cancer Res* 46:4491–4495.

Katano, M., & Torisu, M. (1983) New approach to management for ascites with a streptococcal preparation, OK-432. II. Intraperitoneal inflammatory cell-mediated tumor cell destruction. *Surgery* 93:365–373.

Kavoussi, L. R., Torrence, R. J., Gillen, D. P., Hudson, M. A., Haaff, E. O., Dresner, S. M., Ratliff, T. L., & Catalona, W. J. (1988) Results of 6 weekly intravesical Bacillus Calmette-Guerin instillations on the treatment of superficial bladder tumors. *J Urol* 139:935–940.

Kefford, R. F., Woods, R. L., Fox, R. M., & Tattersall, M. H. N. (1980) Intracavitary adriamycin, nitrogen mustard and tetracycline in the control of malignant effusions: A randomized study. *Med J Aust* 2:447–448.

Kelley, D. R., Haaff, E. O., Becich, M., Lage, J., Bauer, W. C., Dresner, S. M., Catalona, W. J., & Ratliff, T. L. (1986) Prognostic value of purified protein derivative skin test and granuloma formation in patients treated with intravesical Bacillus Calmette-Guerin. *J Urol* 135:268–271.

Kelley, D. R., Ratliff, T. L., Catalona, W. J., Shapiro, A., Lage, J. M., Bauer, W. C., Haaff, E. O., & Dresner, S. M. (1985) Intravesical Bacillus Calmette-Guerin therapy for superficial bladder cancer: Effect of Bacillus Calmette-Guerin viability on treatment results. *J Urol* 134:48–53.

Kemeny, M. M., Battifora, H., Blayney, D. W., Cecchi, G., Goldberg, D. A., Leong, L. A., Margolin, K. A., & Terz, J. J. (1985) Sclerosing cholangitis after continuous hepatic artery infusion of FUDR. *Ann Surg* 202:176–181.

Kemeny, M. M., Goldberg, D., Beatty, J. D., Blayney, D., Browning, S., Doroshow, J., Ganteaume, L., Hill, R. L., Kokal, W. A., Riihimaki, D. U., & Terz, J. J. (1986) Results of a prospective randomized trial of continuous regional chemotherapy and hepatic resection as treatment of hepatic metastases from colorectal primaries. *Cancer* 57:492–498.

Kemeny, N. (1983) The systemic chemotherapy of hepatic metastases. *Semin Oncol* 10:148–158.

Kemeny, N. (1987) Role of chemotherapy in the treatment of colorectal carcinoma. *Semin Surg Oncol* 3:190–214.

Kemeny, N., Cohen, A., Bertino, J. R., Sigurdson, E., Botet, J., & Oderman, P. (1989) Continuous intrahepatic infusion of floxuridine and leucovorin through an implantable pump for the treatment of hepatic metastases from colorectal carcinoma. *Cancer* 65:2446–2450.

Kemeny, N., Daly, J., Oderman, P., Shike, M., Chun, H., Petroni, G., & Geller, N. (1984) Hepatic artery pump infusion: Toxicity and results in patients with metastatic colorectal carcinoma. *J Clin Oncol* 2:595–600.

Kemeny, N., Daly, J., Reichman, B., Geller, N., Botet, J., & Oderman, P. (1987) Intrahepatic or systemic infusion of fluorodeoxyuridine in patients with liver metastases from colorectal carcinoma: A randomized trial. *Ann Intern Med* 459–465.

Kemeny, N., Niedzwiecki, D., Shurgot, B., & Oderman, P. (1989) Prognostic variables in patients with hepatic metastases from colorectal cancer: Importance of medical assessment of liver involvement. *Cancer* 63:742–747.

Kerr, D. J., Harding, M., Farmer, J. G., Amarin, J., Blackie, R. G., Harland, S. J., & Kaye, S. B. (1988) Pharmacokinetics of cis-dichloro-trans-dihydroxy-bis-isopropylamine platinum IV (iproplatinum, CHIP) in patients with normal and impaired renal function and following intraperitoneal administration. *Med Oncol Tumor Pharmacother* 5(3):153–158.

Kerr, I. G., Deangelis, C., Assaad, D. M., & Hanna, S. S. (1987) Drug extravasation along the route of a peritoneal catheter during intraperitoneal chemotherapy. *Cancer* 60:1731–1733.

Khanna, O. P., Chou, R. H., Son, D. L., Mazer, H., Read, J., Nugent, D., Cottone, R., Heeg, M., Rezvan, M., Viek, N., Uhlman, R., & Friedman, M. (1988) Does Bacillus Calmette-Guerin immunotherapy accelerate growth and cause metastatic spread of second primary malignancy? *Urology* 31:459–468.

Khanna, O. P., Son, D. L., Mazer, H., Read, J., Nugent, D., Cottone, R., Heeg, M., Rezvan, M., Viek, N., Uhlman, R., & Friedman, M. (1988) Superficial bladder cancer treated with intravesical Bacillus Calmette-Guerin or Adriamycin: Follow-up report. *Urology* 31:287–293.

Khayat, D., LeeCesne, A., Weil, M., Azar, N., Cour, V., Myle, C. V. T., Auclerc, G., Thill, L., Vallantin, X., Cohen-Aloro, G., Langois, J. C., & Jacquillat, C. (1988) Intra-arterial treatment of hepatic metastases using the 5-fluorouracil, adriamycin, mitomycin C (FAM) chemotherapeutic regiman. *Reg Cancer Treat* 1:62–64.

Killion, J. J., Fan, D., Bucana, C. D., Frangos, D. N., Price, J. E., & Fidler, I. J. (1989) Augmentation of antiproliferative activity of interferon alfa against human bladder tumor cell lines by encapsulation of interferon alfa within liposomes. *JNCI* 81:1387–1392.

Kim, D. K., Watson, R. C., Pahnke, L. D., & Fortner, J. G. (1977) Tumor vascularity as a prognostic factor for hepatic tumor. *Ann Surg* 185:31–34.

Kim, H. H., & Lee, C., (1989) Intravesical mitomycin C instillation as a prophylactic treatment of superficial bladder tumor. *J Urol* 141:1337–1340.

Kim, S., & Howell, S. B. (1987) Multivesicular liposomes containing cytarabine entrapped in the presence of hydrochloric acid for intracavitary chemotherapy. *Cancer Treat Rep* 71:705–711.

Kim, S., Kim, D. J., Geyer, M. A., & Howell, S. B. (1987) Multivesicular liposomes containing ara-C for slow-release intrathecal therapy. *Proc Am Soc Clin Oncol* 6:32.

King, M. E., Pfeifle, C. E., & Howell, S. B. (1984) Intraperitoneal cytosine arabinoside in ovarian carcinoma. *J Clin Oncol* 2:662–669.

Kirmani, S., McVey, L., Loo, D., & Howell, S. B. (1989) Phase 1 clinical trial of intraperitoneal thiotepa in refractory ovarian cancer (abstract). *Proc Am Soc Clin Oncol* 8:157.

Klaase, J. M., Kroon, B. B. R., Benckhuijsen, C., van Geel, A. N., Albus-Lutter, C. E., & Wieberdink, J. (1989) Results of regional isolation perfusion with cytostatics in patients with soft tissue tumors of the extremities. *Cancer* 64:616–621.

Klopp, C. T., Bateman, J., Berry, N., Alford, C., & Winship, T. (1950) Fractionated regional cancer chemotherapy (abstract). *Cancer Res* 10:229.

Knuchel, R., Hofstadter, F., Jenkins, W. E. A., & Masters, J. R. W. (1989) Sensitivities of monolayers and spheroids of the human bladder cancer cell line MGH-U1 to the drugs used for intravesical chemotherapy. *Cancer Res* 49:1397–1401.

Koga, S., Hamazoe, R., Maeta, M., Shimizu, N., Murakami, A., & Wakatsuki, T. (1988) Prophylactic therapy for peritoneal recurrence of gastric cancer by continuous hyperthermic peritoneal perfusion with mitomycin C. *Cancer* 61:232–237.

Komp, D. M., Fernandez, C. H., Falletta, J. M., Ragab, A. H., Humphrey, G. B., Pullen, J., Moon, T., & Shuster, J. (1982) CNS prophylaxis in acute leukemia: Comparison of two methods, a Southwest Oncology Group study. *Cancer* 50:1031–1036.

Kooistra, K. L., Rodriguez, M., & Powis G. (1989) Toxicity of intrathecally administered cytotoxic drugs and their antitumor activity against an intrathecal Walker 256 carcinosarcoma model for meningeal carcinomatosis in the rat. *Cancer Res* 49:977–982.

Koontz, W. W., Jr., Prout, G. R., Jr., Smith, W., Frable, W. J., & Minnis, J. E. (1981) The use of intravesical thio-tepa in the management of non-invasive carcinoma of the bladder. *J Urol* 125:307–312.

Koops, H. S., Beekhuis, H., Oldhoff, J., Oosterhuis, J. W., van der Ploeg, E., & Vermey, A. (1981) Local recurrence and survival in patients with (Clark Level IV/V and over 1.5-mm thickness) Stage I malignant melanoma of the extremities after regional perfusion. *Cancer* 48:1952–1957.

Koops, H. S., & Oldhoff, J. (1983) Hyperthermic regional perfusion in high-risk stage-I malignant melanomas of the extremities. *Recent Results Cancer Res* 86:223–228.

Kottmeier, H. L. (1968) Treatment of ovarian cancer with thiotepa. *Clin Obstet Gynecol* 11:447–448.

Koyama, H., Nishizawa, Y., Wada, T., Kabuto, T., Shiba, E., Iwanaga, T., Terasawa, T., & Wada, A. (1985) Intra-arterial infusion chemotherapy as an induction therapy in multidisciplinary treatment for locally advanced breast cancer. *Cancer* 56:725–729.

Kraft, A. R., Tompkins, R. K., & Jesseph, J. E. (1968) Peritoneal electrolyte absorption: Analysis of portal, systemic venous and lymphatic transport. *Surgery* 64:148–153.

Krementz, E. T. (1983) Chemotherapy by isolated regional perfusion for melanoma of the limbs. *Recent Results Cancer Res* 86:193–203.

Krementz, E. T. (1986) Regional perfusion: Current sophistication, what next? *Cancer* 57:416–432.

Kroon, B. B. R., (1988) Regional isolation perfusion in melanoma of the limbs: Accomplishments, unsolved problems, future. *Eur J Surg Oncol* 14:101–110.

Kroon, B. B. R., van Geel, A. N., Benckhuijsen, C., & Wieberdink, J. (1987) Normothermic isolation perfusion with melphalan for advanced melanoma of the limbs. *Anticancer Res* 7:441–442.

Lafon, P. C., Reed, K., & Rosenthal, D. (1985) Acute cholecystitis associated with hepatic arterial infusion of floxuridine. *Am J Surg* 150:687–689.

Lagasse, L. D., Pretorius, R. G., Petrilli, E. S., Ford, L. C., Hoeschele, J., & Kean, C.

(1981) The metabolism of cis-diamminedichloroplatinum(II): Distribution, clearance, and toxicity. *Am J Obstet Gynecol* 139:791–798.

Lamm, D. L. (1985) Bacillus Calmette-Guerin immunotherapy for bladder cancer. *J Urol* 134:40–47.

Lamm, D. L., Crissman, J. L., Crawford, E. D., Blumenstein, B., Montie, J. E., Scardino, P. T., Grossman, H. B., Stanisic, T., Smith, J. A., & Sarosdy, M. (1989) BCG versus adriamycin intravesical therapy for in situ and papillary transitional cell carcinoma of the urinary bladder: A Southwest Oncology Group study (abstract). *Proc Am Soc Clin Oncol* 8:130.

Lamm, D. L., Stogdill, V. D., Stogdill, B. J., & Crispen, R. G. (1986) Complications of Bacillus Calmette-Guerin immunotherapy in 1,278 patients with bladder cancer. *J Urol* 135:272–274.

Lamm, D. L., Thor, D. E., Stogdill, V. D., & Radwin, H. M. (1982) Bladder cancer immunotherapy. *J Urol* 128:931–934.

Lamm, D. L., Thor, D. E., Winters, W. D., Stogdill, V. D., & Radwin, H. M. (1981) BCG immunotherapy of bladder cancer: Inhibition of tumor recurrence and associated immune responses. *Cancer* 48:82–88.

Laporte, J. P., Godefroy, W., Verny, A., Gorin, N. C., Najman, A., & Ouhamel, G. (1985) Intrathecal mitoxantrone. *Lancet* 2:160.

Lashford, L. S., Davies, A. G., Richardson, R. B., Bourne, S. P., Bullimore, J. A., Eckert, H., Kemshead, J. T., & Coakham, H. B. (1988) A pilot study of ^{131}I monoclonal antibodies in the therapy of leptomeningeal tumors. *Cancer* 61:857–868.

Lathrop, J. C., & Frates, R. E. (1980) Arterial infusion of nitrogen mustard in the treatment of intractable pelvic pain of malignant origin. *Cancer* 45:432–438.

Lathrop, J. C., & Frates, R. E. (1983) The use of nitrogen mustard in the treatment of intractable pelvic pain. *Recent Results Cancer Res* 86:26–32.

Laufman, L. R., Green, J. B., Alberts, D. S., O'Toole, R., Hilgers, R. D., Young, D. C., Lin, F., & Rivkin, S. E. (1986) Chemotherapy of drug-resistant ovarian cancer: A Southwest Oncology Group study. *J Clin Oncol* 4:1374–1379.

Lawrence, W., Jr. (1988) Concepts in limb-sparing treatment of adult soft tissue sarcomas. *Semin Surg Oncol* 4:73–77.

Lawton, F., Blackledge, G., Mould, J., Latief, T., Watson, R., & Chetiyawardana, A. D. (1987) Phase II study of mitoxantrone in epithelial ovarian cancer. *Cancer Treat Rep* 71:627–629.

Lederman, G. S., Recht, A., Herman, T., Osteen, R., Corson, J., & Antman, K. H. (1987) Long-term survival in peritoneal mesothelioma: The role of radiotherapy and combined modality treatment. *Cancer* 59:1882–1886.

Lee, Y-T. M. (1988a) Loco-regional recurrent mesothelioma: II. Non-systemic treatments (1964–1979). *Cancer Treat Rev* 15:105–133.

Lee, Y-T. M. (1988b) Loco-regional primary and recurrent melanoma: III. Update of natural history and non-systemic treatments (1980–1987). *Cancer Treat Rev* 15:135–162.

Lehane, D. E., Byran, R. N., Horowitz, B., DeSantos, L., Ehni, G., Zubler, M. A., Rudolph, L., Aldama-Leubbert, A., Mahoney, D., & Harper, R. (1983) Intraarterial cis-platinum chemotherapy for patients with primary and metastatic brain tumors. *Cancer Drug Deliv* 1:69–77.

Lehti, P. M., Moseley, H. S., Janoff, K., Stevens, K., & Fletcher, W. S. (1986) Improved survival for soft tissue sarcoma of the extremities by regional hyperthermic perfusion, local excision and radiation therapy. *Surg Gynecol Obstet* 162:149–152.

Lembersky, B., Baldisseri, M., Kunschner, A., Seski, J., Zook, D., Hammond, R., Herberman, R., Kowal, C., & Kirkwood, J. (1989) Phase I–II study of intraperitoneal low dose interleukin-2 in refractory stage III ovarian cancer (abstract). *Proc Am Soc Clin Oncol* 8:163.

Lerner, H. J., Schoenfeld, D. A., Martin, A., Falkson, G., & Borden, E. (1983) Malignant mesothelioma: The Eastern Cooperative Oncology Group experience. *Cancer* 52:1981–1985.

Levenback, C., Curtin, J., Rubin, S., Yeh, S., Hoskins, W., Chapman, D., Jones, W., Hakes, T., Markman, M., Reichman, B., & Lewis, J. L., Jr. (1989) A longitudinal study of the distribution of intraperitoneally administered fluids as determined by radionuclide scanning (abstract). *Proceedings of the International Gynecologic Cancer Society* 2:161.

Levin, L., & Hryniuk, W. M. (1987) Dose intensity analysis of chemotherapy regimens in ovarian carcinoma. *J Clin Oncol* 5:756–767.

Levin, V. A., Vestnys, P. S., Edwards, M. S., Wara, W. M., Fulton, D., Barger, G., Seager, M., & Wilson, C. B. (1983) Improvement in survival produced by sequential therapies in the treatment of recurrent medulloblastoma. *Cancer* 51:1364–1370.

Lien, W. M., & Ackerman, N. B. (1970) The blood supply of experimental liver metastases. II. A microcirculatory study of the normal and tumor vessels of the liver with the use of perfused silicone rubber. *Surgery* 68:334–340.

Lin, G., Lunderquist, A., Hagerstrand, I., & Boijsen, E. (1984) Postmortem examination of the blood supply and vascular pattern of small liver metastases in man. *Surgery* 96:517–526.

Linn, R., Klinberg, I. W., & Wajsman, Z. (1989) Persistent acid-fast bacilli following intravesical Bacillus Calmette-Guerin. *J Urol* 141:1197–1198.

Lishner, M., Perrin, R. G., Feld, R., Messner, H. A., Tuffnell, P. G., Elhakim, T., Matlow, A., & Curtin, J. E. (1990) Complications associated with Ommaya reservoirs in patients with cancer: The Princess Margaret Hospital experience and a review of the literature. *Arch Intern Med* 150:173–176.

Litam, J. P., Cabanillas, F., Smith, T. L., Bodey, G. P., & Freireich, E. J. (1979) Central nervous system relapse in malignant lymphomas: Risk factors and implications for prophylaxis. *Blood* 54:1249–1257.

Litterst, C. L., Collins, J. M., Lowe, M. C., Arnold, S. T., Powell, D. M., & Guarino, A. M. (1982) Local and systemic toxicity resulting from large-volume Ip administration of doxorubicin in the rat. *Cancer Treat Rep* 66:157–161.

Litterst, C. L., Torres, I. J., Arnold, S., McGunagle, D., Furner, R., Sikic, B. I., & Guarino, A. M. (1982) Absorption of antineoplastic drugs following large-volume Ip administration to rats. *Cancer Treat Rep* 66:147–155.

Littlewood, T. J., Lydon, A. P. M., & Booth F. (1988) Intraarticular and intraperitoneal administration of etoposide in haematological malignancy. *Cancer Chemother Pharmacol* 21:175.

Loeffler, T., & Freund, W. (1986) Pharmacokinetics of mitoxantrone intraperitoneal (abstract). *Proc Am Assoc Cancer Res* 27:175.

Lopez, J. A., Krikorian, J. G., Reich, S. D., Smyth, R. D., Lee, F. H., & Issell, B. F. (1985) Clinical pharmacology of intraperitoneal cisplatin. *Gynecol Oncol* 20:1–9.

Los, G., Mutsaers, P. H. A., van der Vijgh, W. J. F., Baldew, G. S., de Graaf, P. W., & McVie, J. G. (1989) Direct diffusion of cis-diamminedichloroplatinum(II) in intraperitoneal rat tumors after intraperitoneal chemotherapy: A comparison with systemic chemotherapy. *Cancer Res* 49:3380–3384.

Lotze, M. T., Custer, M. C., & Rosenberg, S. A. (1986) Intraperitoneal administration of interleukin-2 in patients with cancer. *Arch Surg* 121:1373–1379.

Louie, K. G., Ozols, R. F., Myers, C. E., Ostchega, Y., Jenkins, J., Howser, D., & Young, R. C. (1986) Long-term results of a cisplatin-containing combination chemotherapy regimen for the treatment of advanced ovarian carcinoma. *J Clin Oncol* 4:1579–1585.

Lucas, W. E. (1984) Surgical principles of intraperitoneal access and therapy. In S. B. Howell (Ed.), *Intra-arterial and Intracavitary Chemotherapy* (pp. 53–60). Boston: Martinus Nijihoff.

Lucas, W. E., Markman, M., & Howell, S. B. (1985) Intraperitoneal chemotherapy for advanced ovarian cancer. *Am J Obstet Gynecol* 152:474–478.

Lukas, G., Brindle, S., & Greengard, P. (1971) The route of absorption of intraperitoneally administered compounds. *J Pharmacol Exp Ther* 178:562–566.

Lundbeck, F., Bruun, E., Finnerup, B., & Christophersen, I. S. (1988) Intravesical therapy of noninvasive bladder tumors (stage TA) with doxorubicin: Initial treatment results and long-term course. *J Urol* 139:1212–1213.

Lundbeck, F., Mogensen, P., & Jeppesen, N. (1983) Intravesical therapy of noninvasive bladder tumors (stage Ta) with doxorubicin and urokinase. *J Urol* 130:1087–1089.

Lutz, R. J., & Miller, D. L. (1988) Mixing studies during hepatic artery infusion in an in vitro model. *Cancer* 62:1066–1073.

Maatman, T. J., Montie, J. E., Bukowski, R. M., Risius, B., & Geisinger, M. (1986) Intra-arterial chemotherapy as an adjuvant to surgery in transitional cell carcinoma of the bladder. *J Urol* 135:256–260.

Mackintosh, F. R., Colby, T. V., Podolsky, W. J., Burke, J. S., Hoppe, R. T., Rosenfelt, F. P., Rosenberg, S. A., & Kaplan, H. S. (1982) Central nervous system involvement in non-Hodgkin's lymphoma: An analysis of 105 cases. *Cancer* 49:586–595.

McVie, J. G., Rodenhuis, S., Dubbelman, R., Varossleau, F. J., & Ten Bokkel Huinink, W. W. (1987) Clinical pharmacokinetics of intraperitoneal mitoxantrone in ovarian cancer (abstract). *Proc Am Soc Clin Oncol* 6:41.

McVie, J. G., Ten Bokkel Huinink, W., Dubbelman, R., Franklin, H., Van Der Vijgh, W., & Klein, I. (1985) Phase I study and pharmacokinetics of intraperitoneal carboplatin. *Cancer Treat Rev* 12(Suppl. A):35–41.

McVie, J. G., Ten Bokkel Huinink, W. W., Hilton, A., Franklin, H., Wanders, J., & Rodenhuis, S. (1989) Carboplatin and cyclophosphamide in relapsing ovarian cancer patients (abstract). *Proc Am Soc Clin Oncol* 8:161.

Madajewicz, S., Kanter, P., West, C., Bhargava, A., Prajapati, R., Caracandas, J., Avellanosa, A., & Fitzpatrick, J. (1981) Plasma, spinal fluid and organ distribution of cis-platinum following intravenous and intracarotid infusion (abstract). *Proc Am Assoc Cancer Res* 22:176.

Madajewicz, S., West, C. R., Park, H. C., Ghoorah, J., Avellanosa, A. M., Takita, H.,

Karakousis, C., Vincent, R., Caracandas, J., & Jennings, E. (1981) Phase II study-intra-arterial BCNU therapy for metastatic brain tumors. *Cancer* 47:653–657.

Mahaley, M. S., Hipp, S. W., Dropcho, E. J., Bertsch, L., Cush, S., Tirey, T., & Gillespie, G. Y. (1989) Intracarotid cisplatin chemotherapy for recurrent gliomas. *J Neurosurg* 70:371–378.

Malone, J. M., Gershenson, D. M., Carrasco, C. H., Charnsangavej, C., Copeland, L. J., Larson, D. M., Kavanagh, J. J., Edwards, C. L., & Wallace, S. (1987) Intrahepatic infusional therapy for metastatic ovarian carcinoma. *Cancer* 59:1866–1969.

Mantovani, A., Sessa, C., Peri, G., Allavana, P., Introna, M., Polentarutti, N., & Mangioni, C. (1981) Intraperitoneal administration of *Corynebacterium parvum* in patients with ascitic ovarian tumors resistant to chemotherapy: Effects on cytotoxicity of tumor-associated macrophages and NK cells. *Int J Cancer* 27:437–446.

Marans, H. Y., & Bekirov, H. M. (1987) Granulomatous hepatitis following intravesical Bacillus Calmette-Guerin therapy for bladder carcinoma. *J Urol* 137:111–112.

Markman, M. (1985) The intracavitary administration of cytarabine to patients with non-hematopoietic malignancies: Pharmacologic rationale and results of clinical trials. *Semin Oncol* 12(2; Suppl. 3):177–183.

Markman, M. (1986) Intraperitoneal anti-neoplastic agents for tumors principally confined to the peritoneal cavity. *Cancer Treat Rev* 13:219–242.

Markman, M. (1987a) The intracavitary administration of biological agents. *J Biol Response Mod* 6:404–411.

Markman, M. (1987b) Intraperitoneal chemotherapy for malignant disease of the gastrointestinal tract. *Surg Gynecol Obstet* 164:89–93.

Markman, M. (1988) An argument in support of cost-effectiveness analysis in oncology. *J Clin Oncol* 6:937–939.

Markman, M., Cleary, S., Howell, S. B., & Lucas, W. E. (1986) Complications of extensive adhesion formation following intraperitoneal chemotherapy. *Surg Gynecol Oncol* 112:445–448.

Markman, M., Cleary, S., King, M. E., & Howell, S. B. (1985) Cisplatin and cytarabine administered intrapleurally as treatment of malignant pleural effusions. *Med Pediatr Oncol* 13:191–193.

Markman, M., Cleary, S., Lucas, W. E., Weiss, R., & Howell, S. B. (1986) Intraperitoneal chemotherapy employing a regimen of cisplatin, cytarabine and bleomycin. *Cancer Treat Rep* 70:755–760.

Markman, M., Cleary, S., Pfeifle, C. E., & Howell, S. B. (1986) Cisplatin administered by the intracavitary route as treatment for malignant mesothelioma. *Cancer* 58:18–21.

Markman, M., George, M., Hakes, T., Reichman, B., Hoskins, W., Rubin, S., Jones, W., Almadrones, L., & Lewis, J. L., Jr., (1990) Phase 2 trial of intraperitoneal mitoxantrone in the management of refractory ovarian carcinoma. *J Clin Oncol* 8:146–150.

Markman, M., & Howell, S. B. (1985a) Daily intraperitoneal administration of cytarabine in a patient with peritoneal mesothelioma. *Cancer Drug Deliv* 2:285–289.

Markman, M., & Howell, S. B. (1985b) Intrapericardial instillation of cisplatin in a patient with a large malignant effusion. *Cancer Drug Deliv* 2:49–52.

Markman, M., Howell, S. B., Cleary, S., & Lucas, W. E. (1985) Intraperitoneal chemotherapy with high dose cisplatin and cytarabine for refractory ovarian carcinoma and other malignancies principally involving the peritoneal cavity. *J Clin Oncol* 3:925–931.

Markman, M., Howell, S. B., & Green, M. R. (1984) Combination intracavitary chemotherapy for malignant pleural disease. *Cancer Drug Deliv* 1:333–336.

Markman, M., Howell, S. B., Lucas, W. E., Pfeifle, C. E., & Green, M. R. (1984) Combination intraperitoneal chemotherapy with cisplatin, cytarabine, and doxorubicin for refractory ovarian carcinoma and other malignancies principally confined to the peritoneal cavity. *J Clin Oncol* 2:1321–1326.

Markman, M., & Kelsen, D. (1989) Intraperitoneal cisplatin and mitomycin as treatment of malignant peritoneal mesothelioma. *Reg Cancer Treat* 2:49–53.

Markman, M., Reichman, B., Ianotti, N., Hoskins, W., Rubin, S., Jones, W., & Lewis, J. L., Jr. (1989) Phase 1 trial of recombinant tumor necrosis factor administered by the intraperitoneal route. *Reg Cancer Treat* 2:174–177.

Markman, M., Rothman, R., Hakes, T., Reichman, B., Hoskins, W., Rubin, S., Jones, W., Almadrones, L., & Lewis, J. L., Jr. (1990) Second-line cisplatin treatment in patients with ovarian cancer previously treated with cisplatin (abstract). *Proc Am Soc Clin Oncol* 9:155.

Markman, M., Vasilev, S., Howell, S. B., & diZerega, G. S. (1986) Inhibition of peritoneal cavity fibrin deposition induced by the intraperitoneal administration of cisplatin plus cytarabine (abstract). *Clin Res* 34:567.

Markman, M., Weiss, R., Howell, S. B., & Lucas, W. E. (1985) The intraoperative intraperitoneal administration of cisplatin: A case report. *Cancer Drug Deliv* 2:87–90.

Martijn, H., Koops, H. S., Milton, G. W., Nap, M., Oosterhuis, J. W., Shaw, H. M., & Oldhoff, J. (1986) Comparison of two methods of treating primary malignant melanomas Clark IV and V, thickness 1.5 mm and greater, localized on the extremities: Wide surgical excision with and without adjuvant regional perfusion. *Cancer* 57: 1923–1930.

Martijn, H., Oldhoff, J., & Koops, H. S. (1981) Regional perfusion in the treatment of patients with locally metastasized malignant melanoma of the limbs. *Eur J Cancer* 17:471–476.

Martin, J. K., Jr., & Goellner, J. R. (1986) Abdominal fluid cytology in patients with gastrointestinal malignant lesions. *Mayo Clin Proc* 61:467–471.

Martinez-Pineiro, J. A., Leon, J. J., Martinez-Pineiro, L., Jr., Fiter, L., Mosteiro, J. A., Navarro, J., Matres, M. J. G., & Carcamo, P. (1990) Bacillus Calmette-Guerin versus doxorubicin versus thiotepa: A randomized prospective study of 202 patients with superficial bladder cancer. *J Urol* 143:502–506.

Mascharak, P. K., Sugiura, Y., Kuwahara, J., Suzuki, T., & Lippard, S. J. (1983) Alteration and activation of sequence-specific cleavage of DNA by bleomycin in the presence of the antitumor drug cis-diamminedichloroplatinum(II). *Proc Natl Acad Sci USA* 80:6795–6798.

Mavligit, G. M., Benjamin, R., Patt, Y. Z., Jaffe, N., Chuang, V., Wallace, S., Murray, J., Ayala, A., Johnston, S., Hersh, E. M., & Calvo, D. B. (1981) Intraarterial cisplatinum for patients with inoperable skeletal tumors. *Cancer* 48:1–4.

Mavligit, G. M., Charnsangavej, C., Carrasco, C. H., Patt, Y. Z., Benjamin, R. S., & Wallace, S. (1988) Regression of ocular melanoma metastatic to the liver after hepatic arterial chemoembolization with cisplatin and polyvinyl sponge. *JAMA* 260: 974–976.

Mehta, B. M., Glass, J. P., & Shapiro, W. R. (1983) Serum and cerebrospinal fluid distribution of 5-methyltetrahydrofolate after intravenous calcium leucovorin and intra-Ommaya methotrexate administration in patients with meningeal carcinomatosis. *Cancer Res* 43:435–438.

Menashe, D. S., & Jacobs, S. C. (1989) Complications of hypogastric artery cisplatin infusions. *J Surg Oncol* 41:160–164.

Menczer, J., Ben-Baruch, G., Modan, M., & Brenner, H. (1989) Intraperitoneal cisplatin chemotherapy versus abdominopelvic irradiation in ovarian carcinoma patients after second-look laparotomy. *Cancer* 63:1509–1513.

Metzger, U., Laffer, U., Castiglione, M., & Senn, H. J. (1989) Adjuvant intraportal chemotherapy for colorectal cancer—4 year results of the randomized Swiss study (abstract). *Proc Am Soc Clin Oncol* 8:105.

Milazzo, J., Mohit-Tabatabai, M. A., Hill, G. J., Raina, S., Swaminathan, A., Cheung, N. K., Dasmahapatra, K., & Rush, B. F., Jr. (1985) Preoperative intra-arterial infusion chemotherapy for advanced squamous cell carcinoma of the mouth and oropharynx. *Cancer* 56:1014–1017.

Miller, A. B., Hoogstraten, B., Staquet, M., & Winkler, A. (1981) Reporting results of cancer treatment. *Cancer* 47:207–214.

Miller, R. L., Bukowski, R. M., Andresen, S., & Gahbauer, R. (1988) Phase II evaluation of sequential hepatic artery infusion of 5-fluorouracil and hepatic irradiation in metastatic colorectal carcinoma. *J Surg Oncol* 37:1–4.

Mintzer, D. M., Kelsen, D., Frimer, D., Heelan, R., & Gralla, R. (1985) Phase II trial of high-dose cisplatin in patients with malignant mesothelioma. *Cancer Treat Rep* 69:711–712.

Mishina, T., Oda, K., Murata, S., Ooe, H., Mori, Y., & Takahashi, T. (1975) Mitomycin C bladder instillation therapy for bladder tumors. *J Urol* 114:217–219.

Monk, B. J., Surwit, E. A., Alberts, D. S., & Graham, V. (1988) Intraperitoneal mitomycin C in the treatment of peritoneal carcinomatosis following second-look surgery. *Semin Oncol* 15(3; Suppl. 4):27–31.

Morales, A. (1984) Long-term results and complications of intracavitary Bacillus Calmette-Guerin therapy for bladder cancer. *J Urol* 132:457–459.

Morales, A., Eidinger, E., & Bruce, A. W. (1976) Intracavitary Bacillus Calmette-Guerin in the treatment of superficial bladder tumors. *J Urol* 116:180–183.

Morales, A., & Pang, A. S. D. (1986) Prophylaxis and therapy of an experimental bladder cancer with biological response modifiers. *J Urol* 135:191–193.

Mortimer, J. E., Taylor, M. E., Schulman, S., Cummings, C., Weymuller, E., Jr. & Laramore, G. (1988) Feasibility and efficacy of weekly intraarterial cisplatin in locally advanced (stage III and IV) head and neck cancers. *J Clin Oncol* 6:969–975.

Muchmore, J. H., Carter, R. D., & Krementz, E. T. (1985) Regional perfusion for malignant melanoma and soft tissue sarcoma: A review. *Cancer Invest* 3:129–143.

Muggia, F. M. (1989) Overview of carboplatin: Replacing, complementing, and extending the therapeutic horizons of cisplatin. *Semin Oncol* 16(2; Suppl. 5):7–13.

Muggia, F. M., Chan, K., Russel, C., Sehgal, K., Speyer, J. L., Sorich, J., Colombo, N., & Beller, U. (1988) Phase I IP fluorodeoxyuridine (abstract). In *Proceedings of the Second International Conference on Intracavitary Chemotherapy* (p. 35). San Diego: University of California.

Muller, H., Aigner, K. R., & Walther, H. (1989) Isolated pelvic perfusion for nonresectable pelvic tumors: A pilot study. *Reg Cancer Treat* 2:92–97.

Muller, H., Walther, H., & Aigner, K. R. (1988) Regional chemotherapy of lung tumors and metastases. *Reg Cancer Treat* 1:44–49.

Murdock, K. C., Wallace, R. E., White, R. J., & Durr, F. E. (1985) Discovery and preclinical development of novantrone. In C. A. Coltman (Ed.), *The Current Status of Novantrone* (pp. 3–13). New York: Park Row.

Mydlo, J. H., Usher, S. M., Camacho, F., & Freed, S. (1986) Retrospective study of efficacy of intravesical BCG alone in treatment of superficial bladder cancer. *Urology* 28:173–175.

Nakada, T., Akiya, T., Yoshikawa, M., Koike, H., & Kayayama, T. (1985) Intravesical instillation of doxorubicin hydrochloride and its incorporation into bladder tumors. *J Urol* 134:54–57.

Nakajima, T., Harashima, S., Hirata, M., & Kajitani, T. (1978) Prognostic and therapeutic values of peritoneal cytology in gastric cancer. *Acta Cytol* (Baltimore) 22:225–229.

Narsete, T., Ansfied, F., Wirtanen, G., Ramierz, G., Wolberg, W., & Jarrett, F. (1977) Gastric ulceration in patients receiving intrahepatic infusion of 5-fluorouracil. *Ann Surg* 186:734–736.

Nederman, T., & Carlsson, J. (1984) Penetration and binding of vinblastine and 5-fluorouracil in cellular spheroids. *Cancer Chemother Pharmacol* 13:131–135.

Neijt, J. P., Ten Bokkel Huinink, W. W., Van Der Burg, M. E. L., & Van Oosterom, A. T. (1986) Complete remission at laparotomy: Still a gold standard in ovarian cancer? (letter). *Lancet* 1:1028.

Neijt, J. P., Ten Bokkel Huinink, W. W., Van Der Burg, M. E. L., Van Oosterom, A. T., Kooyman, C. D., Van Houwelingen, J. C., & Pinedo, H. M. (1984) Combination chemotherapy with or without hexamethylmelamine in alkylating-agent resistant ovarian carcinoma. *Cancer* 53:1467–1472.

Nervi, C., Arcangeli, G., Badaracco, G., Cortese, M., Morelli, M., & Starace, G. (1978) The relevance of tumor size and cell kinetics as predictors of radiation response in head and neck cancer: A randomized study on the effect of intraarterial chemotherapy followed by radiotherapy. *Cancer* 41:900–906.

Netto, N. R., Jr., & Lemoks, G. C. (1983) A comparison of treatment methods for the prophylaxis of recurrent superficial bladder tumors. *J Urol* 129:33–34.

Niederhuber, J. E., & Ensminger, W. D. (1983) Surgical consideration in the management of hepatic neoplasia. *Semin Oncol* 10:135–147.

Niederhuber, J. E., Ensminger, W., Gyves, J., Thrall, J., Walker, S., & Cozzi E. (1984) Regional chemotherapy of colorectal cancer metastatic to the liver. *Cancer* 53:1336–1343.

Nissenkorn, I., Herrod, H., & Soloway, M. S. (1981) Side effects associated with intravesical mitomycin C. *J Urol* 126:596–597.

Noguchi, S., Miyauchi, K., Nishizawa, Y., Koyama, H., & Terasawa, T. (1988) Management of inflammatory carcinoma of the breast with combined modality therapy including intraarterial infusion chemotherapy as an induction therapy: Long-term follow-up results of 28 patients. *Cancer* 61:1483–1491.

Norrell, H., Wilson, C. B., Slagel, D. E., & Clark, D. B. (1974) Leukoencephalopathy following the administration of methotrexate into the cerebrospinal fluid in the treatment of primary brain tumors. *Cancer* 33:923–932.

Nugent, J. L., Bunn, P. A., Jr., Matthews, M. J., Ihde, D. C., Cohen, M. H., Gazdar, A., & Minna, J. D. (1979) CNS metastases in small cell brochogenic carcinoma: Increasing frequency and changing patterns with lengthening survival. *Cancer* 44: 1885–1893.

Oates, R. D., Stilmant, M. M., Freedlund, M. C., & Siroky, M. B. (1988) Granulomatous prostatitis following Bacillus Calmette-Guerin immunotherapy of bladder cancer. *J Urol* 140:751–754.

Obel, E. B. (1976) A comparative study of patients with cancer of the ovary who survived more or less than 10 years. *Acta Obstet Gynecol Scand* 55:429–439.

Oberfield, R. A. (1983a) Intraarterial hepatic infusion chemotherapy in metastatic liver cancer. *Semin Oncol* 10:206–214.

Oberfield, R. A. (1983b) Intra-arterial infusion in tumors of the pelvis. *Recent Results Cancer Res* 86:15–25.

O'Connell, M. J., Hahn, R. G., Rubin, J., & Moertel, C. G. (1988) Chemotherapy of malignant hepatomas with sequential intraarterial doxorubicin and systemic 5-fluorouracil and semustine. *Cancer* 62:1041–1043.

O'Connell, M., Mailliard, J., Martin, J., Fitzgibbons, R., Nagorney, D., Wieand, H., Tschetter, L., & Krook, J. (1989) A controlled trial of regional intra-arterial FUDR versus systemic 5-FU for the treatment of metastatic colorectal cancer confined to the liver (abstract). *Proc Am Soc Clin Oncol* 8:98.

Ohtani, M., Fukushima, S., Okamura, T., Sakata, T., Ito, N., Koiso, K., & Niijima, T. (1984) Effects of intravesical instillation of antitumor chemotherapeutic agents on bladder carcinogenesis in rats treated with N-buty-N-(4-hydroxybutyl)nitrosamine. *Cancer* 54:1525–1529.

O'Keeffe, F., Lorigan, J. G., Charnsangavej, C., Carrasco, C. H., Richli, W. R., & Wallace, S. (1989) Chemotherapy and embolization via the inferior epigastric artery for the treatment of primary and metastatic cancer. *AJR* 152:378–390.

Oldfield, E. H., Dedrick, R. L., Chatterji, D. C., Yeager, R. L., Girton, M. E., Kornblith, P. L., & Doppman, J. L. (1985) Arterial drug infusion with extracorporeal removal. II. Internal carotid carmustine in the rhesus monkey. *Cancer Treat Rep* 69:293–303.

Ommaya, A. K. (1984) Implantable devices for chronic access and drug delivery to the central nervous system. *Cancer Drug Deliv* 1:169–179.

Ongerboer De Visser, B. W., Romers, R., Nooyen, W. H., van Heerde, P., Hart, A. A. M., & McVie, J. G. (1983) Intraventricular methotrexate therapy of leptomeningeal metastasis from breast carcinoma. *Neurology* 33:1565–1572.

Ostrowski, M. J. (1986) An assessment of the long-term results of controlling the reaccumulation of malignant effusions using intracavitary bleomycin. *Cancer* 57: 721–727.

Ostrowski, M. J., & Halsall, G. M. (1982) Intracavitary bleomycin in the management of malignant effusions: A multicenter trial. *Cancer Treat Rep* 66:1903–1907.

Ottery, F. D., Scupham, R. K., & Weese, J. L. (1986) Chemical cholecystitis after intrahepatic chemotherapy: The case for prophylactic cholecystectomy during pump placement. *Dis Colon Rectum* 29:187–190.

Oye, R. K., & Shapiro, M. F. (1984) Reporting results from chemotherapy trials: Does response make a difference in patient survival? *JAMA* 252:2722–2725.

Ozols, R. F., Corden, B. J., Jacob, J., Wesley, M. N., Ostchega, Y., & Young, R. C. (1984) High-dose cisplatin in hypertonic saline. *Ann Intern Med* 100:19–24.

Ozols, R. F., Grotzinger, K. R., Fisher, R. I., Myers, C. E., & Young, R. C. (1979) Kinetic characterization and response to chemotherapy in a transplantable murine ovarian cancer. *Cancer Res* 39:3202–3208.

Ozols, R. F., Locker, G. Y., Doroshow, J. H., Grotzinger, K. R., Myers, C. E., Fisher, R. I., & Young, R. C. (1979a) Chemotherapy for murine ovarian cancer: A rationale for Ip therapy with adriamycin. *Cancer Treat Rep* 63:269–273.

Ozols, R. F., Locker, G. Y., Doroshow, J. H., Grotzinger, K. R., Myers, C. E., & Young, R. C. (1979b) Pharmacokinetics of adriamycin and tissue penetration in murine ovarian cancer. *Cancer Res* 39:3209–3214.

Ozols, R. F., Ostchegas, Y., Myers, C. E., & Young, R. C. (1985) High-dose cisplatin in hypertonic saline in refractory ovarian cancer. *J Clin Oncol* 3:1246–1250.

Ozols, R. F., Speyer, J. L., Jenkins, J., & Myers, C. E. (1984) Phase II trial of 5-FU administered Ip to patients with refractory ovarian cancer. *Cancer Treat Rep* 68:1229–1232.

Ozols, R. F., & Young, R. C. (1987) Ovarian cancer. *Curr Probl Cancer* 11(2):57–122.

Ozols, R. F., Young, R. C., Speyer, J. L., Sugarbaker, P. H., Green, R., Jenkins, J., & Myers, C. E. (1982) Phase 1 and pharmacological studies of adriamycin administered intraperitoneally to patients with ovarian cancer. *Cancer Res* 42:4265–4269.

Paladine, W., Cunningham, T. J., Sponzo, R., Donavan, M., Olson, K., & Horton, J. (1976) Intracavitary bleomycin in the management of malignant effusions. *Cancer* 38:1903–1908.

Panasci, L. C., Skalski, V., St-Germain, J., Lazarus, P., Shinder, M., & Margolese, R. (1982) Pharmacology and toxicity of Ip streptozotocin in ovarian cancer: A case report. *Cancer Treat Rep* 66:1595.

Pater, J. L., Carmichael, J. A., Krepart, G. V., Fraser, R. C., Roy, M., Kirk, M. E., Levitt, M., Brown, L. B., Wilson, K. S., Shelly, W. E., & Willan, A. R. (1987) Second-line chemotherapy of stage III–IV ovarian carcinoma: A randomized comparison of melphalan to melphalan and hexamethylmelamine in patients with persistent disease after doxorubicin and cisplatin. *Cancer Treat Rep* 71:277–281.

Patt, Y. Z., Boddie, A. W., Charnsanqavej, C., Ajani, J. A., Wallace, S., Soski, M., Claghorn, L., & Mavligit, G. M. (1986) Hepatic arterial infusion with floxuridine and cisplatin: Overriding importance of antitumor effect versus degree of tumor burden as determinants of survival among patients with colorectal cancer. *J Clin Oncol* 4:1356–1364.

Patt, Y. Z., Claghorn, L., Charnsangavej, C., Soski, M., Cleary, K., & Mavligit, G. M. (1988) Hepatocellular carcinoma: A retrospective analysis of treatments to manage disease confined to the liver. *Cancer* 61:1884–1888.

Patt, Y. Z., Mavligit, G. M., Chuang, V. P., Wallace, S., Johnston, S., Benjamin, R. S., Valdivieso, M., & Hersh, E. M. (1980) Percutaneous hepatic arterial infusion of mitomycin C and floxuridine: An effective treatment for metastatic colorectal carcinoma in the liver. *Cancer* 46:261–265.

Patt, Y. Z., Wallace, S., Freireich, E. J., Chuang, V. P., Hersh, E. M., & Mavligit,

G. M. (1981) The palliative role of hepatic arterial infusion and arterial occlusion in colorectal carcinoma metastatic to the liver. *Lancet* 1:349–351.

Payne, R., (1987) Role of epidural and intrathecal narcotics and peptides in the management of cancer pain. *Med Clin North Am* 71:313–327.

Pettavel, J., Gardiol, D., Bergier, N., & Schnyder, P. (1988) Necrosis of main bile ducts caused by hepatic artery infusion of 5-fluoro-2-deoxyuridine: A prospective study of enzymatic, radiologic and histologic changes in 13 patients infused in 1984–1986. *Reg Cancer Treat* 1:83–92.

Peylan-Ramu, N., Poplack, D. G., Pizzo, P. A., Adornato, B. T., & DiChiro, G. (1978) Abnormal CT scans of the brain in asymptomatic children with acute lymphocytic leukemia after prophylactic treatment of the central nervous system with radiation and intrathecal chemotherapy. *N Engl J Med* 298:815–818.

Pfeifle, C. E., Howell, S. B., Abramson, I. S., & Markman, M. (1985) Maintenance of peritoneal cavity function by the intraperitoneal administration of 32 percent dextran 70. *Cancer Drug Deliv* 2:291–303.

Pfeifle, C. E., Howell, S. B., Ashburn, W. L., Barone, R. M., & Bookstein, J. J. (1986) Pharmacologic studies of intra-hepatic artery chemotherapy with degradable starch microspheres. *Cancer Drug Deliv* 3:1–13.

Pfeifle, C. E., Howell, S. B., & Bookstein, J. J. (1985) Pilot study of intra-arterial floxuridine, mitomycin and doxorubicin in combination with degradable starch microspheres to treat primary and metastatic tumors of the liver. *Cancer Drug Deliv* 2:305–311.

Pfeifle, C. E., Howell, S. B., & Markman, M. (1985) Intracavitary cisplatin chemotherapy for mesothelioma. *Cancer Treat Rep* 69:205–207.

Pfeifle, C. E., Howell, S. B., Markman, M., & Lucas, W. E. (1984) Totally implantable system for peritoneal access. *J Clin Oncol* 2:1277–1280.

Piccart, M. J., Abrams, J., Dodion, P. F., Crespeigne, N., Sculier, J. P., Pector, J. C., Finet, C., Nouwijnck, C., Bondue, H., Atassi, G., & Kenis, Y. (1988) Intraperitoneal chemotherapy with cisplatin and melphalan. *JNCI* 80:1118–1124.

Piccart, M. J., Speyer, J. L., Markman, M,. Ten Bokkel Huinink, W. W., Alberts, D., Jenkins, J., & Muggia, F. (1985) Intraperitoneal chemotherapy: Technical experience at five institutions. *Semin Oncol* 12(3; Suppl. 4):90–96.

Pinsky, C. M., Camacho, F. J., Kerr, D., Geller, N. L., Klein, F. A., Herr, H. A., Whitmore, W. F., Jr., & Oettgen, H. F. (1985) Intravesical administration of Bacillus Calmette-Guerin in patients with recurrent superficial carcinoma of the urinary bladder: Report of a prospective, randomized trial. *Cancer Treat Rep* 69:47–53.

Pisani, R. J., Colby, T. V., & Williams, D. E. (1988) Malignant mesothelioma of the pleura. *Mayo Clin Proc* 63:1234–1244.

Piver, M. S., & Baker, T. (1986) The potential for optimal (≤ 2 cm) cytoreductive surgery in advanced ovarian carcinoma at a tertiary medical center: A prospective study. *Gynecol Oncol* 24:1–8.

Piver, M. S., Barlow, J. J., Lele, S. B., Bakshi, S., Parthasarathy, K. L., & Bender, M. A. (1982) Intraperitoneal chromic phosphate in peritoneoscopically confirmed stage I ovarian adenocarcinoma. *Am J Obstet Gynecol* 144:836–840.

Piver, M. S., Lele, S. B., Marchetti, D. L., Baker, T. R., Emrich, L. J., & Hartman, A. B. (1988) Surgically documented response to intraperitoneal cisplatin, cytarabine, and bleomycin after intravenous cisplatin-based chemotherapy in advanced ovarian adenocarcinoma. *J Clin Oncol* 6:1679–1684.

Plaus, W. J. (1988) Peritoneal mesothelioma. *Arch Surg* 123:763–766.

Podratz, K. C., Schray, M. F., Wieand, H. S., Edmonson, J. H., Jefferies, J. A., Long, H. J., Malkasian, G. D., Stanhope, C. R., & Wilson, T. O. (1988) Evaluation of treatment and survival after positive second-look laparotomy. *Gynecol Oncol* 31:9–21.

Poon, M. A., O'Connell, M. J., Moertel, C. G., Wieand, H. S., Cullinan, S. A., Everson, L. K., Krook, J. E., Mailliard, J. A., Laurie, J. A., Tschetter, L. K., & Wiesenfeld, M. (1989) Biochemical modulation of fluorouracil: Evidence of significant improvement of survival and quality of life in patients with advanced colorectal carcinoma. *J Clin Oncol* 7:1407–1418.

Posner, J. B. (1977) Management of central nervous system metastases. *Semin Oncol* 4:81–91.

Prescott, S., James, K., Busuttil, A., Hargreave, T. B., Chisholm, G. D., & Smyth, J. F. (1989) HLA-DR expression by high grade superficial bladder cancer treated with BCG. *Br J Urol* 63:264–269.

Pretorius, R. G., Hacker, N. F., Berek, J. S., Ford, L. C., Hoeschele, J. D., Butler, T. A., & Lagasse, L. D. (1983) Pharmacokinetics of Ip cisplatin in refractory ovarian carcinoma. *Cancer Treat Rep* 67:1085–1092.

Price, R. A., & Johnson, W. W. (1973) The central nervous system in childhood leukemia. I. The arachnoid. *Cancer* 31:520–533.

Pritchard, J. D., Mavligit, G. M., Benjamin, R. S., Patt, Y. Z., Calvo, D. B., Hall, S. W., Bodey, G. P., & Wallace, S. (1979) Regression of regionally confined melanoma with intra-arterial cis-diamminedichloroplatinum(II). *Cancer Treat Rep* 63:555–558.

Pritchard, J. D., Mavligit, G. M., Wallace, S., Benjamin, R. S., & McBride, C. M. (1979) Regression of regionally advanced melanoma after arterial infusion with cisplatinum and actinomycin-D. *Clin Oncol* 5:179–182.

Probert, J. C., Thompson, R. W., & Bagshaw, M. A. (1974) Patterns of spread of distant metastases in head and neck cancer. *Cancer* 33:127–133.

Prout, G. R., Jr., Griffin, P. P., & Daly, J. J. (1987) The outcome of conservative treatment of carcinoma in situ of the bladder. *J Urol* 138:766–770.

Prout, G. R., Jr., Griffin, P. P., Nocks, B. N., DeFuria, D., & Daly, J. J. (1982) Intravesical therapy of low stage bladder carcinoma with mitomycin C: Comparison of results in untreated and previously treated patients. *J Urol* 127:1096–1098.

Prout, G. R., Jr., Koontz, W. W., Jr., Coombs, J., Hawkins, I. R., & Friedell, G. H. (1983) Long-term fate of 90 patients with superficial bladder cancer randomly assigned to receive or not to receive thiotepa. *J Urol* 130:677–680.

Pujade-Lauraine, E., Colombo, N., Namer, N., Fumoleau, P., Monnier, A., Nooy, M. A., Falkson, G., Mignot, L., Bugat, R., Oliveira, C. M. D., Mousseau, M., Netter, G., Oberling, F., Coiffier, B., & Brandely, M. (1990) Intraperitoneal human r-INF gamma in patients with residual ovarian carcinoma at second look laparotomy (abstract). *Proc Am Soc Clin Oncol* 9:156.

Ramaldi, A., Introna, M., Colotta, F., Landolfo, S., Colombo, N., Mangioni, C., & Mantovani, A. (1985) Intraperitoneal administration of interferon-β in ovarian cancer patients. *Cancer* 56:294–301.

Rege, V. B., Leone, L. A., Soderberg, C. H., Coleman, G. V., Robidoux, H. J., Fijman,

R., & Brown, J. (1983) Hyperthermic adjuvant perfusion chemotherapy for stage I malignant melanoma of the extremity with literature review. *Cancer* 52:2033–2039.

Reichman, B., Markman, M., Hakes, T., Hoskins, W., Rubin, S., Jones, W., Almadrones, L., Ochoa, M., Jr., Chapman, D., & Lewis, J. L., Jr. (1989a) Intraperitoneal cisplatin and etoposide in the treatment of refractory/recurrent ovarian carcinoma. *J Clin Oncol* 7:1327–1332.

Reichman, B., Markman, M., Hakes, T., Hoskins, W., Rubin, S., Jones, W., Almadrones, L., Yordan, E. L., Jr., Eriksson, J. H., & Lewis, J. L., Jr. (1990) Intraperitoneal cisplatin and ara-c in refractory ovarian carcinoma: A phase 2 trial. *Proc Am Soc Clin Oncol* 9:158.

Reichman, B., Markman, M., Hakes, T., Kelsen, D., Hoskins, W., Rubin, S., Almadrones, L., Ochoa, M., Magill, G., & Lewis, J. L., Jr. (1989b) Phase 1 trial of concurrent intraperitoneal and continuous intravenous infusion of 5-fluorouracil plus intraperitoneal cisplatin in patients with refractory cancer. *Reg Cancer Treat* 2: 223–228.

Reichman, B., Markman, M., Hakes, T., Kemeny, N., Kelsen, D., Hoskins, W., Rubin, S., & Lewis, J. L., Jr. (1988) Phase 1 trial of concurrent intraperitoneal and continuous intravenous infusion of fluorouracil in patients with refractory cancer. *J Clin Oncol* 6:158–162.

Rettenmaier, M. A., Moran, M. F., Ramsinghani, N. F., Colman, M., Syed, N. A., Puthawala, A., Jansen, F. W., & DiSaia, P. J. (1988) Treatment of advanced and recurrent squamous carcinoma of the uterine cervix with constant intraarterial infusion of cisplatin. *Cancer* 61:1301–1303.

Ridge, J. A., Bading, J. R., Gelbard, A. S., Benua, R. S., & Daly, J. M. (1987) Perfusion of colorectal hepatic metastases: Relative distribution of flow from the hepatic artery and portal vein. *Cancer* 59:1547–1553.

Roboz, J., Jacobs, A. J., Holland, J. F., Deppe, G., & Cohen, C. J. (1981) Intraperitoneal infusion of doxorubicin in the treatment of gynecologic carcinomas. *Med Pediatr Oncol* 9:245–250.

Rosenberg, S. A. (1986) The adoptive immunotherapy of cancer using the transfer of activated lymphoid cells and interleukin-2. *Semin Oncol* 13:200–206.

Rosenshein, N., Blake, D., McIntyre, P. A., Parmley, T., Natarajan, T. K., Dvornicky, J., & Nickoloff, E. (1978) The effect of volume on the distribution of substances instilled into the peritoneal cavity. *Gynecol Oncol* 6:106–110.

Rowlinson, G., Snook, D., Busza, A., & Epenetos, A. A. (1987) Antibody-guided localization of intraperitoneal tumors following intraperitoneal or intravenous antibody administration. *Cancer Res* 47:6528–6531.

Rubin, S. C., Hoskins, W. J., Markman, M., Hakes, T., & Lewis, J. L., Jr. (1988) Long term access to the peritoneal cavity in ovarian cancer patients. *Gynecol Oncol* 33: 46–48.

Rubin, S. C., Hoskins, W. J., Saigo, P. E., Hakes, T. B., Markman, M., Cain, J. M., Chapman, D., Almadrones, L., Pierce, V. K., & Lewis, J. L., Jr. (1988) Recurrence following negative second-look laparotomy for ovarian cancer: Analysis of risk factors. *Am J Obstet Gynecol* 159:1094–1098.

Rubinstein, L. J., Herman, M. M., Long, T. F., & Wilbur, J. R. (1975) Disseminated necrotizing leukoencephalopathy: A complication of treated central nervous system leukemia and lymphoma. *Cancer* 35:291–305.

Runowicz, C. D., Dottino, P. R., Shafir, M. A., Mark, M. A., & Cohen, C. J. (1986) Catheter complications associated with intraperitoneal chemotherapy. *Gynecol Oncol* 24:41–50.

Ryan, J., Weiden, P., Crowley, J., & Bloch, K. (1988) Adjuvant portal vein infusion for colorectal cancer: A 3-arm randomized trial (abstract). *Proc Am Soc Clin Oncol* 7:95.

Safi, F., Bittner, R., Roscher, R., Schuhmacher, K., Gaus, W., & Beger, G. H. (1989) Regional chemotherapy for hepatic metastases of colorectal carcinoma (continuous intraarterial versus continuous intraarterial/intravenous therapy): Results of a controlled clinical trial. *Cancer* 64:379–387.

Samson, M. K., Rivkin, S. E., Jones, S. E., Costanzi, J. J., LoBuglio, A. F., Stephens, R. L., Gehan, E. A., & Cummings, G. D. (1984) Dose-response and dose-survival advantage for high versus low-dose cisplatin combined with vinblastine and bleomycin in disseminated testicular cancer: A Southwest Oncology Group study. *Cancer* 53: 1029–1035.

Sariban, E., Edwards, B., Janus, C., & Magrath, I. (1983) Central nervous system involvement in American Burkitt's lymphoma. *J Clin Oncol* 1:677–681.

Sause, W. T., Crowley, J., Eyre, H. J., Rivkin, S. E., Pugh, R. P., Quagliana, J. M., Taylor, S. A., & Molnar, B. (1988) Whole brain irradiation and intrathecal methotrexate in the treatment of solid tumor leptomeningeal metastases—a Southwest Oncology Group study. *J Neurooncol* 6:107–112.

Savaraj, N., Lu, K., Manuel, V., & Loo, T. L. (1982) Pharmacology of mitoxantrone in cancer patients. *Cancer Chemother Pharmacol* 8:113–117.

Savolaine, E. R., Zeiss, J., Schlembach, P. J., Skeel, R. T., McCann, K., & Merrick, H. W. (1989) Role of scintigraphy in establishing optimal perfusion in hepatic arterial infusion pump chemotherapy. *Am J Clin Oncol* 12:68–74.

Schalhorn, A., Peyerl, G., & Denecke, H. (1988) Pharmacokinetics of 5-fluorouracil during isolated liver perfusion. *Reg Cancer Treat* 1:21–27.

Schellhammer, P. F., Ladaga, L. E., & Fillion, M. B. (1986) Bacillus Calmette-Guerin for superficial transitional cell carcinoma of the bladder. *J Urol* 135:261–264.

Schipper, H., Clinch, J., McMurray, A., & Levitt, M. (1984) Measuring the quality of life of cancer patients: The Functional Living Index—Cancer: Development and validation. *J Clin Oncol* 2:472–483.

Schneider, A., Kemeny, N., Chapman, D., Niedzwiecki, D., & Oderman, P. (1989) Intrahepatic mitomycin C as salvage treatment for patients with hepatic metastases from colorectal carcinoma. *Cancer* 64:2203–2206.

Schouwenburg, P. F., Van Putten, L. M., & Snow, G. B. (1980) External carotid artery infusion with single and multiple drug regimens in the rat. *Cancer* 45:2258–2264.

Scudder, S. A., Brophy, N. A., Jacobs, C. D., Lewis, B. J., Fory, L. W., & Sikic, B. I. (1989) Intraperitoneal carboplatin in ovarian cancer: A phase II trial of the Northern California Oncology Group (abstract). *Proc Am Soc Clin Oncol* 8:162.

Sculier, J. P. (1985) Treatment of meningeal carcinomatosis. *Cancer Treat Rev* 12: 95–104.

Seiter, K., Kemeny, N., Berger, M., Niedzwiecki, D., Chapman, D., Sigurdson, E., Cohen, A., & Oderman, P. (1990) A randomized trial of intrahepatic infusion of FUDR with dexamethasone vs FUDR alone in the treatment of metastatic colorectal cancer (abstract). *Proc Am Soc Clin Oncol* 9:108.

Sekiya, S., Iwasawa, H., & Takamizawa, H. (1985) Comparison of the intraperitoneal and intravenous routes of cisplatin administration in an advanced ovarian cancer model of the rat. *Am J Obstet Gynecol* 153:106–111.

Seltzer, V., Vogl, S., & Kaplan, B. (1985) Recurrent ovarian carcinoma: Retreatment utilizing combination chemotherapy including cis-diamminedichloroplatinum in patients previously responding to this agent. *Gynecol Oncol* 21:167–176.

Shani, J., Bertram, J., Russell, C., Dahalan, R., Chen, D. C. P., Parti, R., Ahmadi, J., Kempf, R. A., Kawada, T. K., Muggia, F. M., & Wolf, W. (1989) Noninvasive monitoring of drug biodistribution and metabolism: Studies with intraarterial Pt-195m-cisplatin in humans. *Cancer Res* 49:1877–1881.

Shapiro, A., Ratliff, T. L., Oakley, D. M., & Catalona, W. J. (1984) Comparison of the efficacy of intravesical Bacillus Calmette-Guerin with thiotepa, mitomycin C, poly I:C/poly-L-lysine and cis platinum in murine bladder cancer. *J Urol* 131:139–141.

Shapiro, W. R., Green, S. B., Burger, P. C., Selker, R. G., VanGilder, J. D., Robertson, J. T., Mealey, J., Ransohoff, J., & Mahaley, M. S. (1987) A randomized comparison of intra-arterial vs intravenous BCNU for patients with malignant glioma (study 8301): Interim analysis demonstrating lack of efficacy for intra-arterial BCNU (abstract). *Proc Am Soc Clin Oncol* 6:69.

Shapiro, W. R., Posner, J. B., Ushio, Y., Chernik, N. L., & Young, D. F. (1977) Treatment of meningeal neoplasms. *Cancer Treat Rep* 61:733–743.

Shapiro, W. R., Young, D. F., & Mehta, B. M. (1975) Methotrexate: Distribution in cerebrospinal fluid after intravenous, ventricular and lumbar injections. *N Engl J Med* 293:161–166.

Shea, M., Koziol, J. A., & Howell, S. B. (1984) Kinetics of sodium thiosulfate, a cisplatin neutralizer. *Clin Pharmacol Ther* 35:419–425.

Sheen, M-C. (1988) Intra-arterial infusion chemotherapy for severely disabled head and neck cancer. *Reg Cancer Treat* 1:59–61.

Shelly, W. E., Starreveld, A. A., Carmichael, J. A., O'Connell, G., Roy, M., & Swenerton, K. (1988) Toxicity of abdominopelvic radiation in advanced ovarian carcinoma patients after cisplatin/cyclophosphamide therapy and second-look laparotomy. *Obstet Gynecol* 71:327–332.

Shenkenberg, T. D., & Von Hoff, D. D. (1986) Mitoxantrone: A new anticancer drug with significant activity. *Ann Intern Med* 105:67–81.

Shepard, K. V., Levin, B., Faintuch, J., Doria, M. I., DuBrow, R. A., & Riddel, R. H. (1987) Hepatitis in patients receiving intraarterial chemotherapy for metastatic colorectal carcinoma. *Am J Clin Oncol* 10:36–40.

Shepard, K. V., Levin, B., Karl, R. C., Faintuch, J., DuBrow, R. A., Hagle, M., Cooper, R. M., Beschorner, J., & Stablein, D. (1985) Therapy for metastatic colorectal cancer with hepatic artery infusion chemotherapy using a subcutaneous implanted pump. *J Clin Oncol* 3:161–169.

Shibata, J., Fujiyama, S., Sato, T., Kishimoto, S., Fukushima, S., & Nakano, M. (1989) Hepatic arterial injection chemotherapy with cisplatin suspended in an oily lymphographic agent for hepatocellular carcinoma. *Cancer* 64:1586–1594.

Shiu, M. H., & Fortner, J. G. (1980) Intraperitoneal hyperthermic treatment of implanted peritoneal cancer in rats. *Cancer Res* 40:4081–4084.

Shiu, M. H., Knapper, W. H., Fortner, J. G., Yeh, S., Horowitz, G., Schnog, J., Guerra,

J., Gould-Rossbach, P., & Ray, C. (1986) Regional isolated limb perfusion of melanoma intransit metastases using mechlorethamine (nitrogen mustard). *J Clin Oncol* 4:1819–1826.

Sigurdson, E. R., Ridge, J. A., & Daly, J. M. (1986) Intra-arterial infusion of doxorubicin with degradable starch microspheres. *Arch Surg* 121:1277–1281.

Sigurdson, E. R., Ridge, J. A., Kemeny, N., & Daly, J. M. (1987) Tumor and liver drug uptake following hepatic artery and portal vein infusion. *J Clin Oncol* 5:1836–1840.

Silberman, A. W. (1982) Surgical debulking of tumors. *Surg Gynecol Obstet* 155:577–585.

Silverberg, E., & Lubera, J. A. (1989) Cancer statistics 1989. *CA* 39:3–20.

Sindram, P. J., Snow, G. B., & Van Putten, L. M. (1974) Intra-arterial infusion with methotrexate in the rat. *Br J Cancer* 30:349–354.

Sirotnak, F. M., Schmid, F. A., & DeGraw, J. I. (1989) Intracavitary therapy of murine ovarian cancer with cis-diamminedichloroplatinum(II) and 10-ethyl-10-deazaaminopterin incorporating systemic leucovorin protection. *Cancer Res* 49:2890–2893.

Slayton, R. E., Creasman, W. T., Petty, W., Bundy, B., & Blessing, J. A. (1979) Phase II trial of VP-16-213 in the treatment of advanced squamous cell carcinoma of the cervix and adenocarcinoma of the ovary: A Gynecologic Oncology Group study. *Cancer Treat Rep* 63:2089–2092.

Smith, J. A., Markman, M., Kelsen, D., Reichman, B., Tong, W. P., Duafala, M. E., & Bertino, J. R. (1989) Phase 1 study of intraperitoneal FUDR and leucovorin (abstract). *Proc Am Soc Clin Oncol* 8:64.

Soloway, M. S. (1980) The management of superficial bladder cancer. *Cancer* 45:1856–1865.

Soloway, M. S. (1984) Intravesical and systemic chemotherapy in the management of superficial bladder cancer. *Urol Clin North Am* 11:623–635.

Soloway, M. S. (1988a) Introduction and overview of intravesical therapy for superficial bladder cancer. *Semin Oncol* 31(3):5–16.

Soloway, M. S. (1988b) Intravesical therapy for bladder cancer. *Urol Clin North Am* 15:661–669.

Soloway, M. S., & Ford, K. S. (1983) Thiotepa-induced myelosuppression: Review of 670 bladder instillations. *J Urol* 130:889–891.

Soloway, M. S., & Murphy, W. M. (1979) Experimental chemotherapy of bladder cancer: Systemic and intravesical. *Semin Oncol* 6:166–183.

Soloway, M. S., & Perry, A. (1987) Bacillus Calmette-Guerin for treatment of superficial transitional cell carcinoma of the bladder in patients who have failed thiotepa and/or mitomycin C. *J Urol* 137:871–873.

Solt, D. B., Hay, J. B., & Farber, E. (1977) Comparison of the blood supply to diethylnitorsamine-induced hyperplastic nodules and hepatomas and to the surrounding liver. *Cancer Res* 37:1686–1691.

Sondak, V., Deckers, P. J., Feller, J. H., & Mozden, P. J. (1981) Leptomeningeal spread of breast cancer: Report of case and review of the literature. *Cancer* 48:395–399.

Speyer, J. L. (1985) The rationale behind intraperitoneal chemotherapy in gastrointestinal malignancies. *Semin Oncol* 12(3; Suppl. 4):23–28.

Speyer, J., Beller, U., Colombo, N., Wernz, J., Muggia, F., & Beckman, E. M. (1987) First line intraperitoneal chemotherapy in advanced ovarian adenocarcinoma—a pilot study. *Proc Am Soc Clin Oncol* 6:113.

Speyer, J. L., Collins, J. M., Dedrick, R. L., Brennan, M. F., Buckpitt, A. R., Londer, H., DeVita, V. T., & Myers, C. E. (1980) Phase I pharmacological studies of 5-fluorouracil administered intraperitoneally. *Cancer Res* 40:567–572.

Speyer, J. L., Sugarbaker, P. H., Collins, J. M., Dedrick, R. L., Klecker, R. W., & Myers, C. E. (1981) Portal levels and hepatic clearance of 5-fluorouracil after intraperitoneal administration in humans. *Cancer Res* 41:1916–1922.

Spratt, J. S., Adcock, R. A., Muskovin, M., Sherill, W., & McKeown, J. (1980) Clinical delivery system for intraperitoneal hyperthermic chemotherapy. *Cancer Res* 40:256–260.

Spratt, J. S., Adcock, R. A., Sherrill, W., & Travathen, S. (1980) Hyperthermic peritoneal perfusion system in canines. *Cancer Res* 40:253–255.

Stagg, R. J., Lewis, B. J., Friedman, M. A., Ignoffo, R. J., & Hohn, D. C. (1984) Hepatic arterial chemotherapy for colorectal cancer metastatic to the liver. *Ann Intern Med* 100:736–743.

Stagg, R., Viele, C., Lewis, B., Ignoffo, R., & Hohn, D. (1985) A comparison of external pumps vs implantable pumps for continuous infusion chemotherapy: Compliance, complications, and costs (abstract). *Proc Am Soc Clin Oncol* 4:265.

Stahelin, H. (1976) Delayed toxicity of epipodophyllotoxin derivatives (VM 26 and VP 16-213), due to a local effect. *Eur J Cancer* 12:925–931.

Stanhope, C. R., Smith, J. P., & Rutledge, F. (1977) Second trial drugs in ovarian cancer. *Gynecol Oncol* 5:52–58.

Stanisic, T. H., Donovan, J. M., Lebouton, J., & Graham, A. R. (1987) 5-year experience with intravesical therapy of carcinoma in situ: An inquiry into the risks of "conservative" management. *J Urol* 138:1158–1161.

Steg, A., Leleu, C., Debre, B., Boccon, G. L., & Sicard, D. (1989) Systemic Bacillus Calmette-Guerin infection, 'BCGitis' in patients treated by intravesical Bacillus Calmette-Guerin therapy for bladder cancer. *Eur Urol* 16(3):161–164.

Stehlin, J. S. (1969) Hyperthermic perfusion with chemotherapy for cancers of the extremities. *Surg Gynecol Obstet* 129:305–308.

Stehlin, J. S., De Ipolyi, P. D., Giovanella, B. C., Gutierrez, A. E., & Anderson, R. F. (1975) Soft tissue sarcomas of the extremity: Multidisciplinary therapy employing hyperthermic perfusion. *Am J Surg* 130:643–646.

Stehlin, J. S., De Ipolyi, P. D., Greeff, P. J., McGaff, C. J., Davis, B. R., & McNary, L. (1988) Treatment of cancer of the liver: Twenty years' experience with infusion and resection in 414 patients. *Ann Surg* 208:23–25.

Stephens, F. O. (1983) Pharmacokinetics of intra-arterial chemotherapy. *Recent Results Cancer Res* 86:1–12.

Stephens, F. O. (1988) Management of gastric cancer with regional chemotherapy preceding gastrectomy—5-year survival results. *Reg Cancer Treat* 1:80–82.

Stephens, F. O. (1989) Advanced breast cancer: Primary intra-arterial induction chemotherapy. *Reg Cancer Treat* 2:5–8.

Stephens, F. O., Tattersall, M. H. N., Marsden, W., Waugh, R. C., Green, D., & McCarthy, S. W. (1987) Regional chemotherapy with the use of cisplatin and doxorubicin as primary treatment of advanced sarcomas in shoulder, pelvis, and thigh. *Cancer* 60:724–735.

Stephens, R. O. (1988) Why use regional chemotherapy? Principles and pharmacokinetics. *Reg Cancer Treat* 1:4–8.

Sterchi, J. M. (1985) Hepatic artery infusion for metastatic neoplastic disease. *Surg Gynecol Obstet* 160:477–489.

Stewart, D. J., Benjamin, R. S., Luna, M., Feun, L., Caprioli, R., Seifert, W., & Loo, T. L. (1982a) Human tissue distribution of platinum after cis-diamminedichloroplatinum. *Cancer Chemother Pharmacol* 10:51–54.

Stewart, D. J., Benjamin, R. S., Zimmerman, S., Caprioli, R. M., Wallace, S., Chuang, V., Calvo, D., Samuels, M., Bonura, J., & Loo, T. L. (1983) Clinical pharmacology of intraarterial cis-diamminedichloroplatinum(II). *Cancer Res* 43:917–920.

Stewart, D. J., Eapen, L., Hirte, W. E., Futter, N. G., Moors, D. E., Murphy, P. C., Irvine, A. H., Genest, P., McKay, D. E., Evans, W. K., Rasuli, P., Peterson, R. A., & Maroun, J. A. (1987) Intra-arterial cisplatin for bladder cancer. *J Urol* 138: 302–305.

Stewart, D. J., Futter, N., Maroun, J. A., Murphy, P., McKay, D., & Rasuli, P. (1984) Intra-arterial cisplatin treatment of unresectable or medically inoperable invasive carcinoma of the bladder. *J Urol* 131:258–260.

Stewart, D. J., Grahovac, Z., Hugenholtz, H., Russell, N. A., Richard, M. T., Benoit, B. G., Riding, M. D., Danjoux, C., & Maroun, J. A. (1987) Intraarterial mitomycin-C for recurrent brain metastases. *Am J Clin Oncol* 10:432–436.

Stewart, D. J., Green, R. M., Mikhael, N. Z., Montpetit, V., Thibault, M., & Maroun, J. A. (1986) Human autopsy tissue concentrations of mitoxantrone. *Cancer Treat Rep* 70:1255–1261.

Stewart, D. J., Leavens, M., Maor, M., Feun, L., Luna, M., Bonura, J., Caprioli, R., Loo, T. L., & Benjamin, R. S. (1982) Human central nervous system distribution of cis-diamminedichloroplatinum and use as a radiosensitizer in malignant brain tumors. *Cancer Res* 42:2474–2479.

Stewart, D. J., Mikhael, N. Z., Nair, R. C., Kacew, S., Montpetit, V., Nanji, A., Maroun, J. A., & Howard, K. (1988) Platinum concentrations in human autopsy tumor samples. *Am J Clin Oncol* 11:152–158.

Stewart, D. J., Wallace, S., Feun, L., Leavens, M., Young, S. E., Handel, S., Mavligit, G., & Benjamin, R. S. (1982) A phase 1 study of intracarotid artery infusion of cis-diamminedichloroplatinum(II) in patients with recurrent malignant intracerebral tumors. *Cancer Res* 42:2059–2062.

Stewart, J. S. W., Hird, V., Snook, D., Sullivan, M., Hooker, G., Courtenay-Luck, N., Sivolapenko, G., Griffiths, M., Myers, M. J., Lambert, H. E., Munro, A. J., & Epenetos, A. A. (1989) Intraperitoneal radioimmunotherapy for ovarian cancer: Pharmacokinetics, toxicity, and efficacy of I-131 labeled monoclonal antibodies. *Int J Radiat Oncol Biol Phys* 16:405–413.

Stiff, P. J., Lanzotti, V. J., & Roddick, J. W. (1983) Prolonged combination chemotherapy for ovarian carcinoma does not increase the rate of surgical complete remissions. *Proc Am Soc Clin Oncol* 2:156.

Stine, K. C., Hockenberry, M. J., Harrelson, J., Miner, D., & Falletta, J. M. (1989) Systemic doxorubicin and intraarterial cisplatin preoperative chemotherapy plus postoperative adjuvant chemotherapy in patients with osteosarcoma. *Cancer* 63:848–853.

Storm, F. K., & Morton, D. L. (1985) Value of therapeutic hyperthermic limb perfusion in advanced recurrent melanoma of the lower extremity. *Am J Surg* 150:32–35.

Stratford, I. J., Adams, G. E., Horsman, M. R., Kandaiya, S., Rajaratnam, E. S., &

Williamson, C. (1980) The interaction of misonidazole with radiation, chemotherapeutic agents, or heat: A preliminary report. *Cancer Clin Trials* 3:231–236.

Stricker, P. D., Grant, A. B. F., Hosken, B. M., & Taylor, J. S. (1987) Topical mitomycin C therapy for carcinoma of the bladder. *J Urol* 138:1164–1166.

Strong, J. M., Collins, J. M., Lester, C., & Poplack, D. G. (1986) Pharmacokinetics of intraventricular and intravenous N,N',N''-triethylenethiophosphoramide (thiotepa) in rhesus monkeys and humans. *Cancer Res* 46:6101–6104.

Sugarbaker, E. V., & McBride, C. M. (1976) Survival and regional disease control after isolation-perfusion for invasive stage I melanoma of the extremities. *Cancer* 37: 188–198.

Sugarbaker, P. H., Cunliffe, W., Belliveau, J. F., DeBruijn, E. A., Graves, T., Mullins, R., Schlag, P., & Gianola, F. (1988) Rationale for perioperative intraperitoneal chemotherapy as a surgical adjuvant for gastrointestinal malignancy. *Reg Cancer Treat* 1:66–79.

Sugarbaker, P. H., Gianola, F. J., Speyer, J. C., Wesley, R., Barofsky, I., & Meyers, C. E. (1985) Prospective, randomized trial of intravenous versus intraperitoneal 5-fluorouracil in patients with advanced primary colon or rectal cancer. *Surgery* 98: 414–421.

Sugarbaker, P. H., Klecker, R. W., Gianola, F. J., & Speyer, J. L. (1986) Prolonged treatment schedules with intraperitoneal 5-fluorouracil diminish the local-regional nature of drug distribution. *Am J Clin Oncol* 9:1–7.

Suhrland, L. G., & Weisberger, A. S. (1965) Intracavitary 5-fluorouracil in malignant effusions. *Arch Intern Med* 116:431–433.

Sulfaro, S., Frustaci, S., Volpe, R., Barzan, L., Comoretto, R., Monfardini, S., & Carbone, A. (1989) A pathologic assessment of tumor residue and stromal changes after intraarterial chemotherapy for head and neck carcinomas: A study of serial sections of the whole surgical specimen. *Cancer* 64:994–1001.

Sullivan, R. D., Jones, R., Jr., Schnabel, T. G., & Shorey, J. (1953) The treatment of human cancer with intra-arterial nitrogen mustard (methylbis(2-bhloroethyl)amine hydrochloride) utilizing a simplified cathether technique. *Cancer* 6:121–134.

Sullivan, R. D., Miller, E., Chryssochoos, T., & Watkins, E., Jr. (1962) The clinical effects of the continuous intravenous and intra-arterial infusion of cancer chemotherapeutic compounds. *Cancer Chemother Rep* 16:499–510.

Surwit, E. A., Alberts, D. S., Crisp, W., Jackson, R. A., Grozea, P. N., & Leigh, S. (1983) Multiagent chemotherapy in relapsing ovarian cancer. *Obstet Gynecol* 146: 613–616.

Swenerton, K. D., Evers, J. A., White, G. W., & Boyes, D. A. (1979) Intermittent pelvic infusion with vincristine, bleomycin, and mitomycin C for recurrent carcinoma of the cervix. *Cancer Treat Rep* 63:1379–1381.

Szabo, G., Pentek, Z., Csernay, L., & Hernadi, T. (1989) Drug distribution in intraarterial chemotherapy of head and neck tumors: Xeroangiographic and scintigraphic studies. *Reg Cancer Treat* 2:16–19.

Tandon, R. N., Bunnell, I. L., & Cooper, R. G. (1973) The treatment of metastatic carcinoma of the liver by the percutaneous selective hepatic artery infusion of 5-fluorouracil. *Surgery* 73:118–121.

Taylor, A., Baily, N. A., Halpern, S. E., & Ashburn, W. L. (1985) Loculation as a contraindication to intracavitary ^{32}P chromic phosphate therapy. *J Nucl Med* 16:318–319.

Taylor, I., Brooman, P., & Rowling, J. T. (1977) Adjuvant liver perfusion in colorectal cancer: Initial results of a clinical trial. *Br Med J* 2:1320–1322.

Taylor, I., Machin, D., Mullee, M., Trotter, G., Cooke, T., & West, C. (1985) A randomized controlled trial of adjuvant portal vein cytotoxic perfusion in colorectal cancer. *Br J Surg* 72:359–363.

Taylor, I., Rowling, J., & West, C. (1979) Adjuvant cytotoxic liver perfusion for colorectal cancer. *Br J Surg* 66:833–837.

Ten Bokkel Huinink, W. E., Dubbelman, R., Aartsen, E., Franklin, H., & McVie, J. G. (1985) Experimental and clinical results with intraperitoneal cisplatin. *Semin Oncol* 12(3; Suppl. 4):43–46.

Thigpen, T., Vance, R., Lambuth, B., Balducci, L., Khansur, T., Blessing, J., & McGehee, R. (1987) Chemotherapy for advanced or recurrent gynecologic cancer. *Cancer* 60:2104–2116.

Thom, A. K., Sigurdson, E. R., Bitar, M., & Daly, J. M. (1989) Regional hepatic arterial infusion of degradable starch microspheres increases fluorodeoxyuridine (FUdR) tumor uptake. *Surgery* 105:383–392.

Tochner, Z., Mitchell, J. B., Harrington, F. S., Smith, P., Russo, D. T., & Russo, A. (1985) Treatment of murine intraperitoneal ovarian ascitic tumor with hematoporphyrin derivative and laser light. *Cancer Res* 45:2983–2987.

Tolley, D. A., Hargreave, T. B., Smith, P. H., Williams, J. L., Grigor, K. M., Parmer, M. K. B., Freedman, L. S., & Uscinska, B. M. (1988) Effect of intravesical mitomycin C on recurrence of newly diagnosed superficial bladder cancer: Interim report from the Medical Research Council Subgroup on Superficial Bladder Cancer (Urological Cancer Working Party). *Br Med J* 296:1759–1761.

Tonak, J., Hohenberger, W., Weider, F., & Gohl (1983) Hyperthermic perfusion in malignant melanoma: 5-year results. *Recent Results Cancer Res* 86:229–238.

Torisu, M., Katano, M., Kimura, Y., Itoh, H., & Takesue, M. (1983) New approach to management of malignant ascites with a streptococcal preparation, OK-432. I. Improvement of host immunity and prolongation of survival. *Surgery* 93:357–364.

Torrence, R. J., Kavoussi, L. R., Catalona, W. J., & Ratliff, T. L. (1988) Prognostic factors in patients treated with intravesical Bacillus Calmette-Guerin for superficial bladder cancer. *J Urol* 139:941–944.

Torti, F. M., & Lum, B. L. (1984) The biology and treatment of superficial bladder cancer. *J Clin Oncol* 2:505–531.

Torti, F. M., Shortliffe, L. D., Williams, R. D., Pitts, W. C., Kempson, R. L., Ross, J. C., Palmer, J., Meyers, F., Ferrari, M., Hannigan, J., Spiegel, R., McWhirter, K., & Freiha, F. (1988) Alpha-interferon in superficial bladder cancer: A Northern California Oncology group study. *J Clin Oncol* 6:476–483.

Trump, D. L., Grossman, S. A., Thompson, G., Murray, K., & Wharam, M. (1982) Treatment of neoplastic meningitis with intraventricular thiotepa and methrotrexate. *Cancer Treat Rep* 66:1549–1551.

Tseng, M. H., & Park, H. C. (1985) Pelvic intra-arterial mitomycin C infusion in previously treated patients with metastatic, unresectable, pelvic colorectal cancer and angiographic determination of tumor vascularity. *J Clin Oncol* 3:1093–1100.

Turner, F. W., Tod, D. M., Francis, G. J., Greenhill, B. J., & Couves, C. M. (1962) The technique for isolation-perfusion of the rat hind limb. *Cancer Res* 22:49–52.

Twardowski, Z. J. (1985) Intraperitoneal therapy in renal failure. *Semin Oncol* 12(3; Suppl. 4):81–89.

Urba, S., & Forastiere, A. A. (1988) Retrobulbar neuritis in a patient treated with intra-arterial cisplatin for head and neck cancer. *Cancer* 62:2094–2097.

Ushio, Y., Posner, J. B., & Shapiro, W. R. (1977) Chemotherapy of experimental meningeal carcinomatosis. *Cancer Res* 37:1232–1237.

Utz, D. C., Farrow, G. M., Rife, C. C., Segura, J. W., & Zinke, H. (1980) Carcinoma in situ of the bladder. *Cancer* 45:1842–1848.

Van De Velde, C. J. H., De Brauw, L. M., Sugarbaker, P. H., & Tranberg, K-G. (1988) Hepatic artery infusion chemotherapy: Rationale, results, credits and debits. *Reg Cancer Treat* 1:93–101.

Van Der Meijden, A. P. M., & DeBruyne, F. M. J. (1988) Treatment schedule of intravesical chemotherapy with mitomycin C in superficial bladder cancer: Short-term courses or maintenance therapy. *Urology* 31(Suppl. 3):26–29.

Van Der Meijden, A. P. M., Steerenberg, P. A., van Hoogstraaten, I. M. W., Kerckhaert, J. A., Schreinemachers, L. M. H., Harthoorn-Lasthuizen, E. J., Hagenaars, A. M., de Jong, W. H., Debruijne, F. M. J., & Ruitenberg, E. J. (1989) Immune reactions in patients with superficial bladder cancer after intradermal and intravesical treatment with Bacillus Calmette-Guerin. *Cancer Immunol Immunother* 28:287–295.

Van Geel, A. N., Van Wijk, J., & Wieberdink, J. (1989) Functional morbidity after regional isolated perfusion of the limb for melanoma. *Cancer* 63:1092–1096.

Van Weelde, B. J., Pauwels, E. K., Jones, B., & Van Oosterom, A. T. (1984) Scintigraphic peritoneography in advanced ovarian malignancies: Its value for chemotherapeutic distribution studies. *Clin Radiol* 35:465–468.

Varney, R. R., Goel, R., VanSonnenberg, E., Lucas, W. E., & Casola, G. (1989) Delayed erosion of intraperitoneal chemotherapy catheters into the bowel: Report of two cases. *Cancer* 64:762–764.

Veenema, R. J., Dean, A. L., Jr., Uson, A., Roberts, M., & Longo, F. (1969) Thiotepa bladder instillations: Therapy and prophylaxis for superficial bladder tumors. *J Urol* 101:711–715.

Vennin, P., Hecquet, B., Poissonnier, B., Fournier, C., Lequint, A., Delobelle, A., & Demaille, M. C. (1989) Comparative study of intravenous and intraarterial cisplatinum on intratumoral platinum concentrations in carcinoma of the cervix. *Gynecol Oncol* 32:180–183.

Venook, A. P., Stagg, R. J., & Lewis, B. J. (1988) Regional chemotherapy for colorectal cancer metastatic to the liver. *Oncology* 2(3):19–26.

Veronesi, A., Zagonel, V., Galligioni, E., Tumolo, S., Barzan, L., Lorenzini, M., Comoretto, R., & Grigoletto, E. (1985) High-dose versus low-dose cisplatin in advanced head and neck squamous carcinoma: A randomized study. *J Clin Oncol* 3:1105–1108.

Vider, M., Deland, F. M., & Maruyama, Y. (1976) Loculation as a contraindication to intracavitary ^{32}P chromic phosphate therapy. *J Nucl Med* 17:150–151.

Vogl, S. E., Pagano, M., Davis, T. E., Einhorn, N., Tunca, J. C., Kaplan, B. H., & Arseneau, J. C. (1982) Hexamethylmelamine and cisplatin in advanced ovarian cancer after failure of alkylating-agent therapy. *Cancer Treat Rep* 66:1285–1290.

Voigt, H. (1988) Impact of regional chemotherapy for melanoma metastases. *Anticancer Res* 8:347–350.

Wadler, S., Egorin, M. J., Zuhowski, E. G., Tortorello, L., Salva, K., Runowicz, C. D., & Wiernik, P. H. (1989) Phase 1 clinical and pharmacokinetic study of thiotepa administered intraperitoneally in patients with advanced malignancies. *J Clin Oncol* 7:132–139.

Wajsman, Z., Dhafir, R. A., Pfeffer, M., MacDonald, S., Block, A., Dragone, N,. & Pontes, J. E. (1984) Studies of mitomycin C absorption after intravesical treatment of superficial bladder tumors. *J Urol* 132:30–33.

Wajsman, Z., McGill, W., Englander, J., Huben, R. P., & Pontes, J. E. (1983) Severely contracted bladder following intravesical mitomycin C therapy. *J Urol* 130:340–341.

Wakefield, T., Eckhauser, F., Strodel, W., & Knol, J. (1984) Colocutaneous fistula complicating Tenckhoff catheter placement for intraperitoneal chemotherapy. *J Surg Oncol* 27:205–207.

Walker, R., Gargan, R., DeLattre, J., Rosenblum, M., & Shapiro, W. (1988) Complications of intra-arterial BCNU in the treatment of malignant glioma (abstract). *Proc Am Soc Clin Oncol* 7:84.

Wallace, S., Chuang, V. P., Samuels, M., & Johnson, D. (1982) Transcatheter intraarterial infusion of chemotherapy in advanced bladder cancer. *Cancer* 49:640–645.

Walton, L. A., Blessing, J. A., & Homesley, H. D. (1989) Adverse effects of intraperitoneal fluorouracil in patients with optimal residual ovarian cancer after second-look laparotomy: A Gynecologic Oncology Group study. *J Clin Oncol* 7:466–470.

Wang, J. J., & Pratt, C. B. (1970) Intrathecal arabinosyl cytosine in meningeal leukemia. *Cancer* 25:531–534.

Ward, B., Mather, S., Shepherd, J., Crowther, M., Hawkins, L., Britton, K., & Slevin, M. L. (1988) The treatment of intraperitoneal malignant disease with monoclonal antibody guided ^{131}I radiotherapy. *Br J Cancer* 58:658–662.

Wasserman, T. H., Comis, R. L., Goldsmith, M., Handelsman, H., Penta, J. S., Slavik, M., Soper, W. T., & Carter, S. K. (1975) Tabular analysis of the clinical chemotherapy of solid tumors. *Cancer Chemother Rep* 6:399–419.

Wasserstrom, W. R., Glass, J. P., & Posner, J. B. (1982) Diagnosis and treatment of leptomeningeal metastases from solid tumors: Experience with 90 patients. *Cancer* 49:759–772.

Weiden, P. L. (1988) Intracarotid cisplatin as therapy for melanoma metastatic to brain: Ipsilateral response and contralateral progression. *Am J Med* 85:439–440.

Weisberger, A. S., Levine, B., & Storaasli, J. P. (1955) Use of nitrogen mustard in treatment of serous effusions of neoplastic origin. *JAMA* 159:1704–1707.

Weiss, G. R., Garnick, M. B., Osteen, R. T., Steele, G. D., Jr., Wilson, R. E., Schade, D., Kaplan, W. D., Boxt, L. M., Kandarpa, K., Mayer, R. J., & Frei, E. T. (1983) Long-term hepatic arterial infusion of 5-fluorouracil for liver metastases using an implantable infusion pump. *J Clin Oncol* 5:337–344.

Welch, J. P., & Donaldson, G. A. (1979) The clinical correlation of an autopsy study of recurrent colorectal cancer. *Ann Surg* 189:496–502.

Werner, A., Diedrich, K., Krebs, D., Bode, U., & Musch, E. (1989) Intraoperative, intraperitoneal chemotherapy in advanced gynecological malignancies: A report on the acceptability of a new therapeutic regimen. *Eur J Gynaecol Oncol* 10(1):13–19.

West, G. W., Weichselbau, R., & Little, J. B. (1980) Limited penetration of methotrexate into human osteosarcoma spheroids as a proposed model for solid tumor resistance to adjuvant chemotherapy. *Cancer Res* 40:3665–3668.

Wharton, J. T., Edwards, C. L., & Rutledge, F. N. (1984) Long-term survival after chemotherapy for advanced epithelial ovarian carcinoma. *Am J Obstet Gynecol* 148:997.

Wheeler, R. H., Baker, S. R., & Medvec, B. R. (1984) Single-agent and combination drug regional chemotherapy for head and neck cancer using an implantable infusion pump. *Cancer* 54:1504–1512.

Wheeler, R. H., Ziessman, H. A., Medvec, B. R., Juni, J. E., Thrall, J. H., Keyes, J. W., Pitt, S. R., & Baker, S. R. (1986) Tumor blood flow and systemic shunting in patients receiving intraarterial chemotherapy for head and neck cancer. *Cancer Res* 46:4200–4204.

Whitmore, W. F., Jr. (1979) Surgical management of low stage bladder cancer. *Semin Oncol* 6:207–216.

Wickes, A. D., & Howell, S. B. (1985) Pharmacokinetics of hexamethylmelamine administered via the Ip route in an oil emulsion vehicle. *Cancer Treat Rep* 69:657–662.

Willemse, P. H. B., De Vries, E. G. E., Oosterhuis, B. E., Aalders, J. G., Bouma, J., Mulder, N. H., & Sleijfer, D. Th. (1989) Intraperitoneal human r-IFN 2 alpha in patients with stage III minimal residual ovarian cancer (abstract). *Proc Am Soc Clin Oncol* 8:155.

Williams, N. N., & Daly, J. M. (1989) Infusional versus systemic chemotherapy for liver metastases from colorectal cancer. *Surg Clin North Am* 69:401–410.

Williams, R. D. (1988) Intravesical interferon alfa in the treatment of superficial bladder cancer. *Semin Oncol* 15(5; Suppl. 5):10–13.

Wilmott, N. (1987) Chemoembolisation in regional cancer chemotherapy: A rationale. *Cancer Treat Rev* 14:143–156.

Wolf, B. E., & Sugarbaker, P. H. (1988) Intraperitoneal chemotherapy and immunotherapy. *Recent Results Cancer Res* 110:254–273.

Wollner, I. S., Walker-Andrews, S. C., Smith, J. E., & Ensminger, W. D. (1986) Phase II study of hepatic arterial degradable starch microspheres and mitomycin. *Cancer Drug Deliv* 3:279–284.

Wolmark, N., Wickerham, D., Rockette, H., Fisher, B., Redmond, C., Potvin, M., Davies, R., Robidoux, A., Wexler, M., Gordon, P., Cruz, A., Lerner, H., Horsely, S., & Prager, D. (1990) Adjuvant therapy of colon cancer with portal vein 5-FU hepatic infusion (abstract). *Proc Am Soc Clin Oncol* 9:105.

Wood, C. B., Gillis, C. R., & Blumgart, L. H. (1976) A retrospective study of the natural history of patients with liver metastases from colorectal cancer. *Clin Oncol* 2:285–288.

Wood, D. P., Streem, S. B., & Levin, H. S. (1988) Nephrogenic adenoma in patients with transitional cell carcinoma of the bladder receiving intravesical thiotepa. *J Urol* 139:130–131.

Yagoda, A. (1987) Chemotherapy of urothelial tract tumors. *Cancer* 60:574–585.

Yamada, K., Bremer, A. M., West, C. R., Ghoorah, J., Park, H. C., & Takita, H. (1979) Intra-arterial BCNU therapy in the treatment of metastatic brain tumor from lung carcinoma: A preliminary report. *Cancer* 44:2000–2007.

Yang, H. M., & Reisfeld, R. A. (1988) Pharmacokinetics and mechanism of action of a doxorubicin-monoclonal antibody 0.2.27 conjugate directed to a human melanoma proteoglycan. *JNCI* 80:1154–1159.

Yap, H-Y., Yap, B-S., Rasmussen, S., Levens, M. E., Hotobagyi, G. N., & Blumenschein, G. R. (1982) Treatment for meningeal carcinomatosis in breast cancer. *Cancer* 49:219–222.

Yap, H-Y., Yap, B-S., Tashima, C. K., DiStefano, A., & Blumenschein, G. R. (1978) Meningeal carcinomatosis in breast cancer. *Cancer* 42:283–286.

Yoshida, S., Tanaka, R., Takai, N., & Ono, K. (1988) Local administration of autologous lymphokine-activated killer cells and recombinant interleukin 2 to patients with malignant brain tumors. *Cancer Res* 48:5011–5016.

Young, R. C., Chabner, B. A., Hubbard, S. P., Fisher, R. I., Bender, R. A., Anderson, T., Simon, R. M., Canellos, G. P., & DeVita, V. T. (1978) Advanced ovarian adenocarcinoma: A prospective clinical trial of melphalan (L-PAM) versus combination chemotherapy. *N Engl J Med* 299:1261–1266.

Young, R. C., Howser, D. M., Anderson, T., Fisher, R. I., Jaffe, E., & DeVita, V. T., Jr. (1979) Central nervous system complications of non-Hodgkin's lymphoma: The potential role for prophylactic therapy. *Am J Med* 66:435–443.

Zakris, E. L., Dewhirst, M. W., Riviere, J. E., Hoopes, P. J., Page, R. L., & Oleson, J. R. (1987) Pharmacokinetics and toxicity of intraperitoneal cisplatin combined with regional hyperthermia. *J Clin Oncol* 5:1613–1620.

Zambetti, M., Gianni, L., Escobedo, A., Pizzetti, P., Spatti, G. B., & Bonadonna, G. (1989) First-line chemotherapy with intraperitoneal cisplatin and intravenous cyclophosphamide in ovarian carcinoma: A preliminary report. *Am J Clin Oncol* 12:118–122.

Zimm, S., Cleary, S., Horton, C. N., & Howell, S. B. (1988) Phase 1/pharmacokinetic study of thioguanine administered as a 48-hour continuous intraperitoneal infusion. *J Clin Oncol* 6:696–700.

Zimm, S., Cleary, S., Lucas, W., Weiss, R., Markman, M., Andrews, P., Schiefer, M. A., Horton, C., & Howell, S. B. (1987) Phase I/pharmacokinetic study of intraperitoneal cisplatin and etoposide. *J Clin Oncol* 47:1712–1716.

Zincke, H., Benson, R. C., Jr., Hilton, J. F., & Taylor, W. F. (1985) Intravesical thiotepa and mitomycin C treatment immediately after transurethral resection and later for superficial (stages Ta and Tis) bladder cancer: A prospective, randomized, stratified study with crossover design. *J Urol* 134:1110–1113.

Zincke, H., Utz, D. C., Taylor, W. F., Myers, R. P., & Leary, F. J. (1983) Influence of thiotepa and doxorubicin instillation at time of transurethral surgical treatment of bladder cancer on tumor recurrence: A prospective, randomized, double-blind, controlled trial. *J Urol* 129:505–509.

Index

Regional Antineoplastic Drug Delivery

Designed by Ann Walston

Composed by G & S Typesetters, Inc.
in Times Roman with Helvetica display type

Printed by The Maple Press Company
on 60-lb. Glatfelter Hi-Brite offset
and bound in Holliston Roxite